5 DAYS TO A
FLATTER
STOMACH

5 DAYS TO A
FLATTER
STOMACH

Beat the Bulge and
Banish Bloating

MONICA GRENFELL

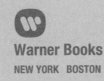

Warner Books

NEW YORK   BOSTON

Neither this nor any other program should be followed without first consulting a health care professional. If you have any special conditions requiring attention, you should consult with your health care professional regularly regarding possible modification of the program contained in this book.

Copyright © 2005 by Monica Grenfell
Previously published in the U.K. by Pan Macmillan

Warner Books
Time Warner Book Group
1271 Avenue of the Americas, New York, NY 10020
Visit our Web site at www.twbookmark.com.

Printed in the United States of America

First Warner Books Edition: May 2005
10 9 8 7 6 5 4 3 2 1

ISBN: 0-446-69536-X
LCCN: 2004116738

Cover photo: Reso/Rex Features

To my sister Shelagh

contents

foreword

Hello, I am Monica Grenfell and this is my 5 DAYS TO A FLATTER STOMACH.

How much do you really want a flatter stomach? Maybe you have been fighting the battle for years as you embark on yet another diet and shell out for gym memberships. Things go well for a while and you lose weight. But your stomach stays stubbornly bloated and uncomfortable, as if some bloat-beast decides to visit, just when you least expected him. How can this happen when you have done all the right things, like exercising and cutting calories?

If all this sounds uncomfortably familiar, you have come to the right place – because I had a serious relationship with the bloat-beast for years. The fact that I beat it is the reason for this book.

Every night for ten years, I squeezed myself into a skintight leotard and leggings and stood in front of 100 pairs of critical eyes as I taught exercise classes. When people are gazing at your stomach, thighs, arms and any other bits which might be flapping in the breeze, night after night, year after year, you learn a few tricks. I dreaded a bloated stomach. My day revolved around making sure it was flat by evening. And this was quite a task. I do not teach fitness these days, but as a qualified nutritionist, I know that the stomach area is the most hated area of the body. You are probably in despair over the bloating, discomfort, and sheer size, in comparison with the rest of your body. I am sure you work hard at it and, believe me, I understand how you feel. After two children (one caesarean) and a couple of stomach operations, not to mention the fact that I am not as young as I was, it is quite a feat to have a flat stomach. But I have, and it is entirely due to this program, which I have developed over many years.

A great body is worth working for. Never believe the doom-mongers who say you can't hope to have a good figure after babies or a flat stomach after forty. You can. The 5-Day program is an amalgamation of all I have learned. I know you are going to be delighted with it and will want to follow the program into the future.

Good luck, and never despair. You can do it!

—Monica Grenfell

introduction

Every woman wants a flat stomach.

Whether or not you champion voluptuous curves, a womanly bottom or a statuesque bosom, nobody wants a big stomach. The success of the first edition of my program prompted this new version, brought up to date but still containing all the elements that made it a hit first time around. A few tricks of the trade, an amazing diet and a good 5-point program to help you manage that stomach for the rest of your life.

So what brings you here? Maybe you have a food intolerance or have been transformed by your pregnancies. Are you bloated beyond what is tolerable? Do you eat because you are happy, or comfort-eat because you are sad? It is a shame to be dissatisfied with your life. You can spend a fortune on designer labels and fill your bathroom with expensive cosmetics, but these just paper over the cracks. If only you felt completely confident about your body, you could pull on a pair of old jeans and everyone would admire you. But if you feel fat or bloated you can dress from head to toe in Chanel and still feel awful inside.

Diets *do* work

Diets don't work if you stop doing them. To explain why you gain weight again after a diet, look at this analogy: a footballer keeps suffering from a knee injury; his playing style is analyzed and he is told that he is running and kicking the wrong way. He goes for an operation and is out of the game for six months. He comes back and plays the same way as before, in the same shoes and on the same surfaces. Guess what — the injury comes back.

If you do the *same* things in the *same* way, you will get the same results. If your old ways made you pile on the pounds, what can you expect if you go back to doing what you did before?

But you have to be sensible. Men don't fall for your fat ratio. Friends can't see your weight. Serving yourself with fat-free alternatives like a second-class citizen while the rest of the family eats the real thing isn't necessary, and on this diet you won't be doing it. I don't want a diet to be so different and quirky from normal life that you draw attention to yourself. For the first time I have taken the stress out of slimming and brought back reality. Reality means food people really want to eat. Reality means not having to spend ten minutes packing your gym bag with equipment and changing into special gear just to go and exercise. Reality means admitting that we don't want to just eat mounds of protein.

5 DAYS — are you SERIOUS?

Of course I am serious!

It takes just five days to settle that stomach and lose excess fluids. In only five days your muscles can be more toned and supple than they have felt for years. The diet is safe and probably healthier than you have eaten for a while. The program takes you into the future and the work will have to be kept up, but the possibilities will delight you:

For example, you have probably been told to do the following:

- eat breakfast like a king, have a filling lunch, and a small dinner
- eat plenty of fruit and vegetables
- eat nothing after 6 p.m.
- start the day with a good breakfast
- nibble on dried fruit for energy
- drink diet drinks instead of the sugary versions
- cut fat
- use low-sugar versions of desserts and sweets.

But on the 5-Day program you will do the following:

- eat four small snacks during the day
- eat most food after 6 p.m.
- eat normal-fat foods, like butter and cheese
- avoid fruit and few vegetables during the day
- have no dried fruit, except a few prunes or apricots in the evening
- eliminate carbonated and diet drinks
- use no artificial sweeteners.

Those are some big changes!

Yes, but you will love them. The biggest blocks to starting something new are fear, skepticism and idleness. Fear that doing something new will disrupt your routine, skepticism because you have tried so many things and they didn't work, and idleness – well, we are all idle about something. Suddenly a year has gone by and you realize you never made that telephone call, wrote that letter or started that diet. But what's the bottom line in all this? Having a flatter stomach. It's why you bought this book. You want it more than anything else, so don't let a few old habits get in the way.

The Grenfell Philosophy

Feeling happy and confident about your figure is your pathway to success. I truly believe this. People who struggle to be slim, even if they profess not to care, are rarely happy and confident inside. They will often try to buy their way to happiness, with designer labels, extravagant shoes and expensive beauty treatments.

Being is more important than *having*. My philosophy is that beauty is the entire effect, and all your clothes and make-up are nothing if you feel fat and unhealthy. Start with the underneath. Don't eat food that clogs your insides and don't pollute yourself with cigarettes and alcohol. What you are is more important than what you have, and if you are healthy, fit and glowing with confidence, you will attract people to you whether or not you are wearing designer clothes or drive a smart car.

And don't you want to give yourself an edge over others? It is not about looking like a celebrity or trying to copy your best friend. It is about presenting the best version of yourself. My simple 5-point program will help you to achieve this. It will help you to remind yourself of your goals and revisit them constantly. This is not about me telling you what to do or what to think; it is about *you* telling yourself what to do and think. You set your own goals and you decide how you are going to achieve them. The Grenfell program simply gives you the framework.

I devised the Grenfell philosophy from mastering my own mind–body connection. It has enabled me to stay the same weight and shape for more than thirty years. I can truly say that I have never gained a pound or increased my vital statistics in all that time, and this certainly is not down to luck. Like you, I have to work at it. Like you, I need a proper diet. I have my bottom line, which I repeat frequently—that I want to be healthy and confident. The reassuring point for you, I hope, is that it has not made me self-obsessed or manic about my weight—far from it. Once you have your program in place you will not be obsessed, because your body takes care of itself. You learn that beauty is the entire effect, nobody can see your weight and it is OK to have that chocolate.

It all starts here

You are probably a diet veteran and already have your eagle eyes peeled for the get-out clause. You're probably used to the scenario where you lose those vanity pounds only to have them creep back on in the following days or weeks. Well, this is not a fad and it isn't a con. This is the 5-Day promise:

You will:
- banish bloating
- lose inches from waist and abdomen
- increase energy
- sleep better
- be more confident
- feel healthier.

And the plus-side is that so much of this plan re-introduces foods that die-hard dieters thought were off the menu for good. Butter and cheese. Rice pudding and potatoes. Seasoned slimmers will have already shrunk from the idea, convinced that their weight will soar overnight and the whole thing will end in tears. But give it five days and I promise you'll be amazed.

Tried and tested

I have been putting clients through this program for years, but for the purposes of this book, I asked another 200 women who wanted to lose weight to try the plan.

None of the testers had any idea what the program was aiming to achieve, only that I was trialling a diet-and-exercise plan for a book. They all kept diaries for me, as I was interested not only in changes in their weight and improvement, but also in whether the meals worked, whether their families enjoyed them, and whether they could find the foods easily. It is no good suggesting a regime which puts people to endless trouble, or stipulating food that can't be taken to work.

The detailed responses of some of the team are contained in the next section (page 10). However, the diaries showed that:

- all the testers lost weight
- all the testers felt noticeably and pleasingly slimmer
- all the testers had managed to give up any laxatives and stomach medicines they had been taking for flatulence, and were thrilled at how calming the diet was
- all the testers said they could happily stick with the regime
- all the testers said they were pleased and relieved to be able to eat "proper" food again – such as butter, eggs and cheese
- nobody disliked the diet in any way.

I believe I cannot go better than the evidence of those 200 volunteers who put themselves through my 5-Day program and my grateful thanks go out to them all. Don't be skeptical. If such results can be achieved in only five days, think what you can achieve in a month!

Is This You? The Reasons People Don't Stick with a Diet

1 I don't see results quickly enough

Crash diets used to be a quick way of losing weight and cheering yourself up, but they gave you false hopes. If you lost six pounds in your first week, a three-pound loss the following week felt like failure. Only one and a half pounds lost the next time and you were nearly suicidal. Never mind that this is perfectly standard weight loss – to you it felt like total standstill. Why be hungry, you reasoned, when nothing was happening? Focusing only on the downside, you forgot that six pounds off was good in itself. "I should have lost fifteen pounds by now!" you moaned. Well, cheer up. The beauty of this diet is real inch loss. Seeing and feeling a real difference is a major psychological boost, which is why the 5-Day program is so popular. This is not a crash diet, but the results are swift.

2 I used to be slim and be able to lose weight easily – now I'm older, the weight just won't go. What's happening? It's not fair!

Look, I want to be ten years younger too, but it isn't going to happen. We all did a lot of things differently when we were younger and, yes, now you have to run hard just to stay in the same place. But I promise that once you get into the 5-Day program you'll be slim, vigorous and glad you made the effort.

Never mind what your age is, or that you've just had your fourth baby, or that operation. Even if you are eighty, you can lose weight. If you take hormone tablets or have thyroid malfunction or you are Type 1 diabetic, you can still lose weight. Feeling that you are somehow a "special" case is a cop-out. It's easy to blame circumstances for your not losing weight. If you start finding reasons why life used to be so much better, you'll never stop.

3 I reach a plateau and there doesn't seem to be any point

Yes, there is. Every scientific test I have ever seen has found that under strict conditions people lost weight at a continuous rate. There is no such thing as a plateau and everyone can lose the amount of weight they wish to lose – as long as they have excess body fat.

So take heart – you can lose those last ten pounds with the Grenfell Maintenance program.

4 I have to make one meal for myself and another for the rest of the family
My meals can be enjoyed by everyone. I don't use any low-calorie or low-fat alternatives, although some recipes are adapted to reduce thoughtless and liberal use of
fattening ingredients. There is no need to treat yourself as a second-class citizen just
because you want to lose weight. We all appreciate quality, and that means real
butter, cheese and cream. As a guide, ask yourself what kind of dessert you would
give to a guest. The lowest-calorie version or the richest? Many of the meals on this
diet are standard favorites, which old and young alike can enjoy.

5 I feel hungry all the time
On this diet, you will be eating five or six times a day. The secret is to eat *small
amounts of food regularly.* Ever woken at 3 a.m. feeling bright and wide awake,
only to fall back to sleep and crawl out of bed in the morning feeling terrible? This
is classic low blood sugar. My mid-evening snack gives you a restful sleep and you'll
wake feeling refreshed.

6 I feel washed out and tired
Calorie-reduced or low-carbohydrate diets can make you very tired, as you are not
putting any energy into your body. The 5-Day diet is completely different, because
the staple daytime foods, while being light, are carbohydrates, and your daily intake
of carbohydrate will be quite high. Your main meal, in particular, will be based on
starchy carbohydrates, so you will feel energetic on the program.

7 I feel bloated on all that fruit and fiber
Fruit is *meant* to fill you. It contains fiber and water and it flushes out your system
wonderfully. If you have a constipation problem, eat fruit. However, there is a
problem, because much fruit contains sorbitol, a natural sweetener that can cause
bloating. If your stomach feels lovely and flat in the morning but bloated by early
evening and you have been eating fruit, you've found the culprit. On this diet, you
will simply shift all that wonderful fruit to the evening, out of harm's way.

How You Will Succeed

You are probably dying to know the secret by now. Well, hold on a little longer while I explain the simple methods to achieving that flatter stomach by the end of the week.

Limited Choice

If your kitchen usually looks like a harvest festival the minute you start a new diet, with your fridge overflowing with fruits and vegetables, you are already on the way to failure. Stocking up on a huge variety of foods is a key to overeating, and scientific research has shown that when you are presented with a wide variety of choices, you will eat more.

The 5-Day program presents you with a few key foods as part of a greatly simplified diet. Any time you are faced with those all-you-can-eat buffets, go for just two or three items rather than a bit of everything.

Going Low – Sodium, That Is

Don't get me wrong – your body needs sodium. It's a mineral that helps the body regulate blood pressure. It's also needed for muscle and nerve function. But you only need around 500–1,000mg a day and that is the amount in one smoked sausage!

And if you want to put a stop to that bothersome bloating, don't dread the bread — the problem is more likely to be sodium overload. You see, salt stimulates the taste buds, making you want an opposing taste. The more salt you have, the more likely you are to want sugar. The more sugar you eat, the more you will crave something sharp, bitter or salty. Simple food takes some getting used to, but it is surely better to have a basic diet, say, during the week, if you know it will help to stop cravings. Save your all-out sushi night for a treat.

However, before you ban savory foods, be aware that there is also a lot of salt in sweet foods like chocolate and cereals.

There is more sodium in a cup of Raisin Bran cereal (486mg) than in a cup of dry-roasted peanuts (9mg).

So go and check out your pantry and read food labels: a low-sodium food contains no more than 140mg of sodium per serving.

These are all high in sodium:

- table salt
- seasonings that contain salt (celery salt, onion salt, etc.)
- canned vegetables in salt water
- olives, pickles, and pickled foods
- regular canned soups
- breads and rolls with salt toppings
- potato chips, corn chips, pretzels, saltines, salty crackers, salted popcorn
- salty or smoked meats (bacon, corned beef, frankfurters, ham, deli meats, sausage, canned or smoked meats)
- salty or smoked fish (anchovies, herring, sardines)
- processed cheese, cheese spreads
- salted nuts
- peanut butter
- ketchup, chilli sauces, meat extracts, monosodium glutamate, mustard, soy sauce, Worcestershire sauce
- antacids containing sodium
- baking-soda toothpaste.

Don't worry if this appears to leave very little. You can still be creative with spices, herbs and even wine and spirits to give your meals flavor.

Exercise That Works

Nobody ever felt worse for exercising properly. The danger is setting yourself too high a goal and going at it like a bull at a gate. If you start on day one promising yourself an hour's aerobics and 500 sit-ups every day, you'll feel a failure when you can't keep it up.

My exercise plan combines a bit of the old, in crunches and standard sit-ups, with something new and exciting: a stretch band. This band is simple and easy to use, and the results it gives are astounding. The exercise section of this book includes a few fantastic exercises that incorporate the stretch band and absolutely anybody can do them.

Do remember that your midsection forms a circle. When you exercise the abdominal muscles on their own, two-thirds of that circle sits idle. On the Grenfell program, you will be toning your waist muscles and your back to provide a strong, balanced center, lifting and toning your entire torso for pleasing posture and a tight tummy.

Posture stretches

However good your muscles are, however slim you have become, if you stand and sit badly your stomach will hang out. Every day of the program includes posture stretches to maintain good body alignment, which alone can make you appear inches slimmer.

No Substitutes for the Best Foods

"I can't believe I'll be eating butter!" said one of my testers. "My last diet banned cheese completely," said another, adding that a lifetime without her favorite cheese-and-pickle sandwich wouldn't be worth living. I agree with her.

Nobody sticks with a menu plan stuffed with "healthy alternatives." The alternatives are often not healthy; in fact, they're often crammed so full of additives that the list of ingredients takes up half the packaging. Yes, my diet insists on actual butter, sour cream, cheese and eggs, but it is a long way from being a high-protein diet. When the nation has been existing on a diet of chips, hot dogs, sweets, ice cream, and pizza, washed down with beer or carbonated drinks, this diet is the healthiest food some people will have eaten for years.

Two-speed diet choice

My diet plan comes in two speeds:

1 **The 5 Days to a Flatter Stomach program** – this can be done for any five days you like, whenever you want a flatter stomach fast

2 **The Lifetime Maintenance program** – the full, 5-step program to ensure you lose weight, achieve a better shape *and* keep your flatter stomach for good!

The 5-Day program is very specific about what to eat and it guarantees fantastic results. The Lifetime Maintenance program offers slightly more choice and features my 5-point program to remind you of your commitment. If you want to know how to keep up the good eating habits you've learned, this diet offers more meal choices and variety, and you'll continue to lose weight steadily as long as you have excess body fat.

Half the battle is your determination. Going for a few walks and eating smaller meals isn't hard, but if you hate going out and love your local takeout it's going to take a shift in attitude. *Do* keep at it. No woman was ever sorry she lost a spare tire. No woman ever looked back wistfully to her "fat" days, when she felt bloated and self-conscious.

Good luck!

Success Stories

How the Testers Got On

My whole weight-loss concept is so different from most diets, I wanted to put a team of testers through it. Not just to prove it worked, but to see if it was practical. After all, it's no good embarking on a punishing regime that makes the whole family suffer, and nobody wants a sandwich lunch that is soggy by the time you get to work. I put the word out and literally thousands of women came forward to test the plan.

I chose a cross-section of people. A couple of women wanted to lose at least 30 lbs., several testers reported few problems with their weight, but despair with their stomachs after having babies, and the majority simply wanted to lose about seven to ten pounds and tone up their muscles. They all kept diaries for me, and I'm delighted to report that their results exceeded my wildest expectations. Here is a selection of their verdicts:

Irene Norton, forty-two, a medical secretary, is married with four teenage children

I had to let you know straight away how completely thrilled I was with the program. I needed to lose more than 15 lbs., but I find conventional diets too long-winded and not really practical for long-term use.

At first I thought "Five days! I'll believe it when I see it!" but because my problem has always been psychological – I suppose I want instant success or I get disheartened – this was the perfect plan for me because I *felt* so much slimmer by the end of just three days, and that spurred me on.

I had to give up the diet for a long weekend because we went away for a wedding, and I realized how awful I'd always felt before. It's the bloating, I think, and when your stomach's wrong you feel wrong all over. I've now gone back to it and I'm following the Maintenance program, which is incredibly do-able. I have lost twelve pounds in five weeks, gone down a dress size and, most important, lost a lot of inches.

To tell the truth, I couldn't care less about what the scales say, I'm more interested in how my clothes look, and my eldest daughter said yesterday that I looked ten years younger now I'm back to cinching in my waist with a nice belt.

I'm really proud of my figure now, the diet's wonderful and I'll keep on the maintenance plan for good. It's nice to have someone spell it all out for you.

Maria Telling, eighteen, is single and a sociology student

The exercises worked best for me. I'm very untoned as I'm lazy about exercise, and my stomach had got quite flabby. Knowing there was only five minutes of exercising meant that I wasn't reluctant to do it, and although it wasn't easy, it worked! I was particularly thrilled with the flex bands. I haven't used anything like them before and I'm quite addicted now! They have toned up my lower stomach quite beautifully in just eight weeks.

I didn't believe that you could do so much without going to an aerobics class for an hour at a time, but I can honestly say that after five days I had an entirely different shape. I hold myself better too and I think that's made a huge difference.

As far as the food was concerned, it was perfect. I'm sharing an apartment that has an ancient oven and only two electric burners, so anything complicated was obviously out. I've also got no money! I spent far less on this diet than I usually do eating at the dining hall at college, and my favorite meal was the spaghetti bolognese, because we could all share it, and it was affordable, which was brilliant.

Siobhan Everitt, thirty, is married with three children under age five

The 5-Day program is great. I wanted to lose about 7 lbs. and have tried a lot of diets, but this is the first one I'd stuck with. I suffer from irritable bowel syndrome, which blows me out, but with this diet I was so much better, with less flatulence and grumbling feelings. I think it was because it wasn't just fruit, fruit, fruit, which always makes me feel quite empty.

I have to work hard at keeping slim, because with three children there's always the wrong food around and you're always making something. I'll have a Milky Way Bar in the afternoon because I'm starving, then I'll think, "Oh, I can't have any tea because I ate that chocolate," so I'm hungry again in the evening and eat cookies, so really it's a lot of junk I'm eating. And so it goes on.

With the program, the food is so enjoyable. I felt I learned a lot, too. It was nice to eat more in the evening after so many years of being told you can't eat after 6 p.m. The most valuable part about it was the philosophy of the Maintenance program. Monica asked many questions that hit the nail right on the head. Having a "bottom line" and a 5-point program to follow meant I could remind myself continually of what this was all about and bring myself back in line. I liked that.

I loved the avocado. I have never eaten one before and I thought, "I'm not sure about this, but it's on the diet," so I tried it with the shrimp. It was wonderful!

I'm carrying on with the program from now on. I lost four pounds and my stomach seems so much slimmer. I won't eat the old way ever again.

Gillian Jaworsky, thirty-five, is an actress, married without children
I admit to being obsessed with my body, and I notice every inch on it. My husband and I entertain, so I was a bit worried I'd either be stuck with awful casseroles or have to give up the diet altogether when we entertained. How wrong I was! I could eat sour cream!

I'm an intermittent, picky eater. I also binge, then starve for days because I feel wretched. I suppose it is because I am in the theater and my job means looking good and it's quite stressful. I tend to go for three days being good, then I eat a square of chocolate and think I might as well eat the bar. Then I hate myself so much that I have two or three slices of cake which I don't even like. Anyway, I was thrilled to be chosen to test this diet, and even more thrilled to say that I ate quite normally – which for me seemed a lot – and I even lost two pounds in the five days. I think it's marvellous.

Anita Frame, forty-three, a dental receptionist, is a divorced mother of four
I am very particular about how I look, especially as I've joined a dating agency recently and am going out on dates now. I needed to tone up a bit and probably should lose about 15 lbs.

On my other diets, if I went out I was terrified of having butter with my bread and I'd ask for any sauce to be left off. On this diet I felt completely liberated! It is difficult to describe, but I now just say yes to everything. As I have learned to eat small amounts and not worry that I'll never eat a square meal again, I feel as if all the tension of a diet has gone. I've done the program now for three weeks and have lost 7 lbs, and the best thing is that I feel I'm not on a diet at all.

I invited one man I met over to my house and cooked him the spaghetti. It took me about ten minutes from start to finish, and he was going mad, saying how fantastic it was and that I must have been slaving away for hours. I didn't say anything!

I just can't believe how toned I feel, and how flat my stomach is. I was really, really unsure of it when I was chosen, but now I'm telling all my friends about the 5-Day program. My children can all eat exactly the same as me, and as one of my daughters has a small weight problem I'm pleased that she's losing weight too.

Helen Foster, thirty-one, a unit-trust dealer, lives with her partner
My oatmeal breakfast filled me up so much I almost didn't need my mid-morning snack every day, but I ate it and wasn't so hungry by lunchtime.

I haven't much of a weight problem, but I'm always holding my stomach in. I didn't think I'd get used to the amount of food – usually I tend to pig out when I get home from work as I'm so hungry, but eating a mid-afternoon snack ended that. I could happily go right through until dinner and eat far less.

I work at home these days, so I got a kitchen timer and put that to go off every hour. I just got on the floor and did twenty sit-ups. It sounds stupid, but it worked for me. I think they made all the difference.

By day five I was definitely into the swing of it. At first, I thought I would be hungry, especially at night, but it seems that I am eating most of the time and I lost three pounds by day four. I'm sure I've lost about one inch off my hips! On day five I put on a skirt that I always use for testing my size and it felt quite roomy! Great!

I'm starting the Lifetime Maintenance program next week. I'm off during the holiday and I'll want to have a few drinks and sweet things but not undo all the good work I've just done. Then when I come back

I will start the 5-Day program again, in case I've gained any weight. I know I do not have a real figure problem, but my stomach drives me crazy and I'm always hiding it. This program is just wonderful; I think I'll stay on it for good.

Marian Crawford, thirty-seven, is a housewife with three children

I'm tall, 5 foot 10, and I was stick-thin before I had my children. It's my stomach that gets me down, I feel I can take in tucks at the sides! Having children has been like blowing up a balloon, keeping it there all Christmas and letting it down again – it never goes back to what it was before, does it?

I needed to tone up, and I found the best help were the stomach exercises. I've also got terrible insides. I'm on the go all day with the children and two new little puppies and I don't often eat much from breakfast to 3 p.m. I was taking vitamins because I was tired, then laxatives because I was constipated! On this diet, I managed to give all that up. My stomach was less grumbly and felt much flatter, and I am pleased I don't have all that bloatedness now.

I never used to drink much water or eat much fruit, and now I will, as it has sorted my problems out. I looked at the diet sheet and thought, "There's so much food – I'll put on weight," but I lost four pounds and wasn't hungry for a minute. I'll definitely keep it up.

Janet and Simon Ashworth, fifty-one and fifty, are both nurses and have grown-up children

Janet: We decided to go on the diet together, for support. Simon wouldn't have gone on any of my other diets (which I'm always starting!) because he says the food's too finicky, but when he saw omelettes, mashed potatoes and roast chicken his eyes lit up.

I must admit I was a bit skeptical about cooking something in butter, but after all the years I've been on these low-fat spreads, good old butter was fantastic. I know you can't have too much of it, but somehow knowing that you're eating the real thing makes you go easy on it anyway. It was like pure gold!

I suppose I'm quite overweight – about 35 lbs. – and Simon's the same. I've been dieting for as long as I can remember, but what puts me off is calculating the portions, measuring each out and then piling on the vegetables because you can't eat again for hours. This diet was such common sense because you just eat small amounts of everything.

My dress is much looser around my stomach, and think I have lost two inches, although I can't have, can I? I'm going onto the Maintenance program to lose the rest of my excess weight.

Simon: I joined Janet to support her, thinking I'd hate it. In fact, I've lost weight too. I feel much, much smaller in my abdomen, and far healthier. I don't know what it is, but I'm really bouncing around now. I've managed to give up my morning chocolate bar with no cravings, and no diet's ever got me to do that!

It was hard at first, I'll admit, to look at a small plate of salad or a couple of spoons of veggies, but you soon want much less. I tried to eat a piece of fish and three potatoes today and had to stop after two of them, I was so full. I think this diet's the best thing that's ever happened to us.

Louise Cordas, twenty-seven, is married with one child and another on the way

I actually lost 60 lbs. to get married! Then I put it back on, got pregnant and thought there wasn't any point. After Matthew was born I knew I should diet, but in the back of my mind was the thought that I knew we wanted two children quite close together and there wouldn't be any point in dieting only to get pregnant again.

I started the diet just before I got pregnant with this one, so obviously I've given it up for a bit, but I'll start it straight away after the birth. I totally believe in this diet. The main thing I like is that I can give my little boy anything I have to eat, which isn't the case with some fancy diet books with all their exotic menus. I never felt hungry, but I knew that if I did I could eat some yogurt and not even think about it. I loved the pasta primavera. All the ingredients were in the local supermarket, so I got everything there and didn't have to traipse around.

I can't wait to go back on it and lose all this weight again.

Dee Whittaker, forty-eight, a beauty therapist, is widowed with two adult daughters

Although I'm a beauty therapist, I've let myself go since my husband died. I always used to play badminton and swim, but the exercise went out of the window last year when I felt so depressed. My weight soared and I couldn't do anything about it.

I've lost four pounds. I actually found the posture section most revealing – I didn't realize until I caught sight of myself in a shop window that I was slouching so badly. My neck was all scrunched up and my chest seemed to sink into my stomach! I think about it all the time now, and it's made my stomach hold itself in and look controlled, which has made me look more confident, my friend tells me.

I thought that exercising several times a day would be a chore, but I started to look forward to it. It was like sending myself on a course. I felt I had homework to do several times a day. Each page of the diet was like Monica talking to me and encouraging me, and the best encouragement was that she said it had worked for her.

I don't want to stop. I feel I can adapt the ideas for myself now, which is the idea of the Maintenance program. It starts off seeming weird with all that mashed potato, rice pudding and bananas, and I didn't think I'd like live and active yogurt cultures. I'd recommend this diet plan to anyone of any age. My stomach's much, much flatter, and I've got my confidence back.

Sally Pallister, twenty-three, is single and works as a journalist for a women's magazine

My life is one mad rush from the beginning of the day to the end, and I go for long hours without eating. Then when I do, it's all the wrong things. I grab a sandwich or stop at one of the local bistros for a snack, which is usually a burger, then I feel completely blown up for hours. I also sit at my computer for up to six hours without a break, and my bottom was spreading. I weighed about ten pounds too much and my figure was a disgrace for someone my age, but I thought, "What can I do?"

If I hadn't been chosen to be a tester I wouldn't have bothered with a diet, but when I saw the meals all written out for me it took away the responsibility and I said yes straight away. I'm so glad I did.

What I liked was the simplicity. I'm always out, and my new toaster which I've had for six months is still in its cellophane! I haven't got a freezer either, so it wouldn't have been any good if I'd needed frozen stuff. The food was the type anyone would like, with no preparation if you didn't want to, and it really worked. After the five days I was four pounds lighter, but I felt really quite svelte. My stomach had lost all its hugeness and I didn't need to hold it in all the time. I did do the exercises too, which was an effort for me as I hate exercise, but as it was only a few minutes here and there I thought it was worth it. Frankly, I didn't think so few exercises would make a difference, but they have.

I've decided to stick with the 5-Day plan every Monday to Friday and as I have a hectic social life at weekends I'll do my own thing then, though I won't go overboard. I'd recommend the diet to any of my friends.

Molly Agnew, seventy-eight, is a retired principal

I've always been careful about my appearance, and just because I'm retired it doesn't mean I've given up. I still like to wear tailored clothes and I have a lot of Christmas engagements this year.

My stomach's more delicate than it used to be and I can't take too many spices or fiber. But the diet worked. The yogurt was somehow calming and I've just worn a skirt I haven't fitted into for ten years!

Linda Thompson, forty, an assistant recruitment manager, is married with two children

I'm a lifelong member of the diet club, and at the moment I'd say my weight's stable. I lost three pounds on the diet, and my friend who did it with me lost a good inch off her stomach in only five days!

I really liked the fact that when I started work at 9 a.m. I knew I didn't have to wait long before I could have a snack. I couldn't have gone on until lunchtime.

We eat late in the evening at home, so I saved the main meal until 9 p.m. I particularly liked the fish content of the diet and I would definitely stick with the Maintenance plan. I think it was a great diet, and it was nice to see results so quickly. I never knew there were so many additives in the diet foods I'd been eating – it really makes you think, doesn't it?

Getting Down to it

Why Is Your Stomach So Big?

It does not take a medical degree to work out why your midsection has gotten out of control:

1 you are constantly bloated
2 you are overweight
3 you are constipated
4 your muscles need toning
5 your posture is terrible

Before you feel too overwhelmed about yourself, let us look at each of these in turn, and see how the 5-Day program can help:

1 You Are Constantly Bloated

This topic is really a book in itself. Has bloating always been a problem or is it worse these days? If it *has* gotten worse, do we know why? Did our grandparents suffer from bloated stomachs? And what does the term mean anyway?

By way of clearing the decks, I asked a gastroenterologist what was meant by bloating. It is most commonly intestinal gas, which causes pressure and distension of the abdomen. Women complain of it more than men do, but on investigation it was usually found that the amount of intestinal gas was the same in both sexes—women simply felt worse about it and had lower tolerance to it.

Our grandparents might well have experienced this sort of discomfort, but were accustomed to it. We are more sensitive these days, and certainly years ago people did not assume that gas and flatulence were in any way unusual. Added to this is the fact that women wore corsets or foundation garments that held everything in place so a distended stomach could be hidden. I am not talking about the Dark Ages, by the way. I was handed a small stretchy thing called a "roll-on" as soon as I reached adolescence, its purpose being to hold in my young-womanly tummy. It was assumed that you needed one!

Hormonal shifts do make us feel bloated. The hormone estrogen rises in mid-cycle as the lining of your womb prepares for a fertilized egg, and it has violent and sudden shifts when you experience menopause. This can make you feel full and uncomfortable. As hormonal bloating is automatically resolved after a few days, I will not expound on the subject here.

Foods to Avoid During the Day

High-fiber products

Whole grains are wonderful and every diet should have them. However, they are sources of insoluble fiber – fiber that passes through the gut whole. Bran, the outer husk of grain, which acts as nature's "scrubbing brush" can cause irritation to the gut, and the bacteria it produces in the large bowel ferment and produce gas. I suggest you avoid these altogether on your important days. You can either do the 5-Day program any time you have something important coming along, or adopt it for just twenty-four hours simply by omitting all high-fiber foods.

Insoluble fiber is also found in:

- nuts
- rice
- strawberries
- many breakfast cereals.

Fruit

All fruit contains fructose (a form of carbohydrate) and it appears that most people have a limit to the amount of fructose they can absorb. When this limit is exceeded, fructose enters the colon, where it ferments, producing gas.

Some fruits also contain sorbitol, which is a natural sugar alcohol. Sorbitol-containing fruits seem to produce more gas than other fruits. Fruits containing sorbitol include:

- apples
- pears
- cherries
- plums
- peaches.

The juice of these fruits also contains sorbitol.

From a practical point of view, it makes sense to cut back on fruit if you suffer from a lot of gas. Do not eliminate fruit, but watch portion size. On the 5-Day program, I encourage you to eat fruit in the evening to get maximum benefit from its laxative properties.

However, the reason some fruits are not suitable for those in search of a flat stomach is their fiber content. Apples have a lovely soluble fiber (see page 26) called pectin in their flesh – but their skin is insoluble fiber and will pass through your body as it came in. All fruit skins can be a problem, so *peel that fruit!* Though you must eat some skins if you become debilitatingly constipated.

Cruciferous vegetables

Cruciferous vegetables are a family of vegetables that includes cabbage, Brussels sprouts, cauliflower, broccoli, and kale. You do not need me to tell you that these can cause a great deal of gas, so you will not eat them at all when you are doing the 5-Day program.

Of course, when you are "between programs" or at any other time to suit yourself, feel free to eat as many of these wonderful vegetables as you like.

Legumes

Legumes include peas, all kinds of beans, lentils and sweetcorn. Legumes contain protein, they are low in fat and high in fiber because the outer skin or shell cannot be broken down by the body, so it passes through the system whole.

The reputation of beans and lentils as gas producers goes before them. It is said that if you eat them often enough, the effect ceases. Frankly, I would rather not take the risk.

Carbonated drinks

Do not have them! They are full of gas that simply passes through to your insides.

Food Intolerances

Irritable bowel syndrome (IBS) and food intolerances in general have been big news for the last few years. I am astounded that they have taken such a hold when one never used to hear of them. I can vaguely remember an aunt saying that cucumber "didn't agree with her" or my mother complaining that coffee gave her heartburn, but that was it. Being intolerant of food was not a concept anyone would have recognized, unless of course they were seriously ill or suffering from a major food allergy. Celiac disease, extreme hypersensitivity to gluten (found in wheat, oats, barley and rye), was also well documented. But sensitivity to bananas, bread or fish?

I am sure many people will dispute this. There are always exceptions to a rule and somebody will have suffered intolerances fifty years ago. Nonetheless, I go back to what I have just said: perfectly healthy, functioning adults would not have phoned before a dinner party to say they could not eat wheat or dairy foods, neither would they demand that a restaurant adapt their meals to accommodate their food intolerances. Not if they were otherwise healthy. The "done" thing was to shift the food round your plate, eat what you could manage and disguise what you had left under a few vegetables. We have all struggled through a plate of something disgusting swimming in grease, but that's life.

This diet makes much of foods to avoid or leave for another time, but this is a trick to help you achieve the best results. I am not suggesting that you have an intolerance simply because some foods tend to make you flatulent, constipated, or bloated.

When you read the next section, about chemicals and additives, you will see what I mean. I certainly believe that what we eat can cause havoc in our insides, but that is due to the massive amounts of chemicals added. When you read my directions on eating, swallowing, chewing and so on, you will see that eating habits are another questionable area.

Poor eating habits can have the most devastating effects on your system, including foul gas, bloating, excess acid and a feeling of fullness hours after a meal. It is no wonder that you immediately blame what you have just eaten, and as wheat is in so many foods, and is eaten in some form or another for breakfast (cereal, toast), lunch (sandwiches) and snacks (cake), it is not surprising that wheat is a contender when we look for something to blame.

But who eats "wheat"? Bread has other things in it, a sandwich has a filling, pasta and pizzas have toppings, and what about the salads that come on the side or the fruit juice you drank after your breakfast toast?

In other words, wheat alone may not be to blame.

I would look instead to soy flour and to emulsifiers. Soy, while perfectly good and nutritious, can be an allergen. It can cause a mild reaction in some people, who will probably not even know that they have a sensitivity to it. Personally, I stay a million miles from anything with soy, not because I am allergic but because I dislike the inevitable effects. It has a tendency – I will put it no stronger than that – to cause bloating.

Then there are emulsifiers. Look at the wrapping on a standard loaf of commercial bread and I bet you will see these listed along with the soy. There are other things too, and often the loaves are treated to make them last a week or even two. If your loaf is still fresh after a week, avoid it next time. Proper bread should be stale after a couple of days.

My answer is to make your own bread. A recipe for this is on page 113. It might seem cumbersome, but if you make several loaves you can slice and freeze them, ready to take slices as you need them. You also have the satisfaction of eating your own wholesome bread, free from soy flour and artificial additives.

I would be foolish to suggest that food intolerances do not exist. Of course they do. But please try my simple practical measures before dismissing whole food groups from your diet.

Chemicals and Additives

Let me read to you the list of ingredients from a standard pack of own-brand white rolls from a leading supermarket:

Wheat flour, Water, Vegetable oil, Hydrogenated vegetable oil, Salt, Yeast, Dextrose, Emulsifiers: Sodium stearyl-2-lactylate and Mono- and diacetyl tartaric acid; Esters of mono- and diglycerides of fatty acids, Soy flour, Flour treatment agent: L-ascorbic acid

The pack also states that the rolls "may contain traces of nuts and sesame seeds."

Now, I have been making my own bread for years, and to make white bread I use unbleached wheat flour, yeast, water, salt, sugar and a little butter or olive oil. Nothing else. The bread keeps a couple of days; if I want to keep it longer, I freeze it.

I am still struggling to understand why bought bread needs all those extra ingredients. I found similar ingredients in cereal bars, cakes, soups, packet sauces and so on. The lists would take several pages of this book. The real question is: what are all these additives doing to your body?

The additives are harmless. They would not be there if they weren't. But I truly believe it has been forgotten that our bodies were designed to process food and water. We are incredibly robust and, with a good amount of stomach acid, thorough chewing, and a stable environment (which means not too much stress), our digestive system can tackle most things. But emulsifiers? Hydrogenated fat, which is known to be a health risk? And while I am at it, what are traces of nuts and sesame seeds doing in white bread?

Additives are thought of as essential because without them our food spoils more quickly. They prevent hardness and rancidity, and in many cases additives inhibit the growth of salmonella and other harmful bacteria. It would be wrong to condemn them out of hand, but few people realize that many additives cause the discomfort of abdominal bloating and flatulence, and the bulging stomach we simply can't hold in.

In the quest for a lower-fat diet, manufacturers have had to come up with increasingly creative ways of cutting calories in their products without sacrificing the taste. They have found that adding seaweeds, gums, and emulsifiers, not to mention pumping vast quantities of air into everything, makes low-calorie food look and taste like the real thing. The drawbacks have been twofold: first, you tend to eat twice as much because you think you are getting half the calories, and second, the additives have unfortunate effects on your digestive system.

Don't get me wrong. I am not a health freak. I just don't see the point in the tiny calorie saving if the results are unflattering and embarrassing.

Here is a list of the most commonly used additives which have a laxative effect, and therefore cause a grumbling and flatulent stomach:

Sorbitol (E420), isomalt, mannitol and xylitol
These are all sweeteners known to have a laxative effect in high doses. Found in sausages, soft-scoop ice cream, sugar-free jams and sugar-free sweets. In susceptible individuals, especially children, the effects can include a distressingly distended stomach.

Sorbitol is also present quite naturally in fruits like apples, cherries, peaches, apricots and plums, and these fruits seem to produce more gas than other fruits do.

Carrageenan (E407)
This seaweed-derived product is an emulsifier, and is used to thicken and improve consistency. Found in quick-setting jellies, milkshakes, biscuits, pastries, meat pies, sausages and instant

mousses. Has caused concern for its laxative effect, especially in children.

Guar gum (E412), gum arabic (E414) and xanthan gum (E415)

Can cause flatulence through a laxative effect. Found in salad dressings, soft cheese, coleslaw, canned vegetables, processed cheese, pickles, wine, beer, candy, and yogurts that don't contain live and active cultures.

Air

Not an additive in the accepted sense, but included here because it is added to some foods to give them volume. For example, ice creams and some desserts are often pumped with air to lower the calorie content weight for weight. Taking in extra air is the primary cause of intestinal gas, so avoid foods which boast very low calories if possible.

The list of lesser-known and little-used additives which can cause intestinal problems is long, but they need not concern us here as my object is to alert you to the most commonly used additives that you are likely to find in your everyday foods. I must stress that these substances are not harmful in small doses, but remember that the average diet – especially a slimming diet – will probably include not just one or two, but many of these products every day. The cumulative laxative effect of these additives is something you are unlikely to be aware of. Personally, I see little virtue in giving up natural sugar only to eat large quantities of chemical alternatives.

I am not including a comprehensive discussion of additives because I believe the solution is obvious – eat fresh food. The 5-Day program uses only fresh ingredients to make meals that are easy to prepare and even easier to freeze, so if you want convenience food, you can have home-cooked, additive-free meals at hand at any time.

How You Eat

Next on the list of causes of bloating is how you eat. This is one of the most important factors, and the point where I start to sound like a mother nagging her children for not minding their table manners. Even if you eliminate the wrong foods, all your good intentions will be thwarted if you eat the wrong way. Being on the program means you have to be rigid about how you eat.

Eat slowly

When you see food and smell it, your digestive juices start flowing. This is stomach acid, ready to break down your food and churn it into a paste before sending it on its way through your gut. If you see food and gulp it down, huge lumps of food enter the stomach, which has to grind away on overtime to turn it into something manageable. The result: gas!

Another cause of flatulence is swallowed air. You swallow air when you:

- talk or laugh while eating
- chew gum
- slurp drinks
- slurp food
- take too much food onto your fork – you know it's too much when it is hard to fit it all in your mouth!

The result is great pockets of air that blow you out.

It's hard to train yourself to eat slowly, especially if you were brought up in a household where everyone ate as fast as possible, or if you missed out on second helpings if you ate too slowly. It's hard if you have only a short time in which to eat. But if you eat more slowly and carefully you will feel full much sooner, and this way you will eat less.

Chew food to a paste

A typical fast eater is usually loading the fork or spoon before the previous mouthful has been swallowed. This is a bad habit. Train yourself to put your cutlery down between mouthfuls and not pick it up again until you have swallowed. The digestive system works to a series of signals, the first of which is the chewing action. This alerts your system that something is on its way and stomach acids are set in motion. The longer you chew, the more acid is produced and, of course, the food is then nicely broken up, can be digested with the minimum of fuss and you feel fine.

Chewing something once or twice before swallowing does not allow your stomach to get ready. It also has to deal with lumps of food rather than a nice paste. Chewing will go a long way to *significantly* reducing bloating.

Try not to eat under stress

Easier said than done, but if a problem is gnawing away at you, or you are sitting at the dinner table fuming after an argument, the effects on your digestion can be pretty unpleasant. The most common complaint is painful stomach cramps an hour or two after eating. An attack of nerves, such as on an important date or before an interview, can also bring on the most dreadful spasms. If you are under stress during a meal, avoid meat and poultry and stick with fish and mashed root vegetables like potatoes and carrots.

Do not leave long gaps between meals

Leaving more than three hours between small meals means that you not only get hungry and are therefore likely to eat more than you need, but also that the build-up of stomach acid and emptiness can lead to indigestion. Think in terms of a yawning, empty hole in your stomach which suddenly receives a massive amount of food all at once, and probably too quickly. Being on a diet that restricts you to only three meals a day means that you will tend to make the most of every meal. Your stomach, which has been empty for up to five waking hours, then has to cope with a lot of food in one go. If you have a bloating problem, you should not go for more than three hours during the day without something in your stomach.

2 You Are Overweight

Fat settles all too easily on your stomach. This is because the mid-section gets the least movement. Everyday routine forces us to move our arms and legs, but the midsection needs specific movements. Sitting for hours on end is the real killer. But even if you get up and get moving and get a good fat-loss diet going, you could still fail to crack this problem. This is because the key is not what you eat, but why you eat.

Eating when bored

You might not feel bored as you rush around with ten things to do at once, but you can be bored of being busy. Food becomes a time-filler.

So don't fill time with eating! There are so many other productive things to do. If your office or home is a mess, either clear out a drawer or tidy a room. Rather than eat, take the fridge apart and enjoy chucking out leftovers. You will have the benefits of a job done as well as the saving of your waistline.

Eating the wrong things

There's no such thing as a bad food. Not even chocolate or chips or sugar or butter. There are only bad diets. Eating chocolate is not a problem and chips are not fattening. What *is* wrong is a diet of chips, then chocolate, followed by lots of alcohol. Day after day! A balance of small amounts of every-thing is the key to a great body and flat stomach.

Not using up your food intake

Fat settles because your food is surplus to require-ments. Nothing very earth-shattering there. So why not make your requirements greater? Exercise doesn't have to be manic fitness; it can be move-ment of any kind. Each time you move, you raise your calorie-burn rate slightly. If you move fast, you raise it more. If you put in a bit more effort, like going from walking on the treadmill to the StairMaster, the calorie-burn rises again, taking you from one calorie a minute burned to four calories a minute, and so on. This is a terrific way to increase calorie requirements rather than eating less.

Metabolic rates and eating too little

If you lay In bed doing absolutely nothing all day, you would still need energy to keep you alive. This is called your Basal Metabolic rate (BMR). In fact, you can work out your BMR – how much energy your body uses just keeping you alive – like this.

For women	For men
Weight in lbs x 0.409	**Weight in lbs x 0.425**

This tells you the number of calories you use per HOUR. So, for a woman weighing 130lbs: BMR = 130 x 0.409 = 53.17. Let's just call that 53 calories. Multiply by 24 to find BMR in a day: 53 x 24 = 1,272 calories.
To work out your added energy requirements, you need a bit of honesty and realism.

- If you are sedentary, sit more than 5 hours a day in an office or at home, multiply this number by 1.2 So, 1,272 x 1.2 = 1,526
- If you are fairly active, walk more than 30 minutes to work or take the children to school and spend more than 3 hours day on your feet, multiply by 1.3 So, 1,272 x 1.3 = 1,653
- If you are moderately active, exercise aerobically for more than an hour five times a week and have an active lifestyle, x 1.4
- If you are very active, have a job walking or moving about all day, or otherwise exercise more than 6 hours a week x 1.5

Eating too little actually makes you gain weight in the long run. Your body is programed to preserve life, so if your food intake is reduced your metabolism slows down. It doesn't happen overnight. If you remember that nature's job is to preserve life at all costs, you can understand why cutting out food in order to stay slim just does not work. If you have consistently irregular eating patterns, your metabolism will slow down to preserve your fat supplies as your body adjusts to try to keep you alive as long as possible. Eating little and often serves the dual purpose of preventing weight gain and keeping your metabolism ticking away happily at a moderate rate, so that the calories you have taken in are burnt efficiently.

Lack of will power

You might say you lack will power. This is an easy cop-out to save your brain from having to exert any reasonable psychological force. Lack of will power happens when you see a diet as something unpleasant and avoidable. But isn't getting up night after night to a crying baby unpleasant? Or going to do a job you don't like every day? But you would do it, and this proves that you *do* have will power in some form.

The 5-Day program is a daily reminder of the things you have to do because they become part of your life. Rather than being on a diet, you are on a program that will fit beautifully into your life. You won't lack will power ever again.

Beating Cravings

The greater the distance between wanting something and having it, the less likely you are to end up with it. This is how credit cards work. If you had to go home and get the cash every time you saw a fabulous outfit, you would only buy a fraction of what you see. A credit card turns wanting into having all too quickly, and this is how cravings take hold.

If you crave chocolate and have it lying around – well, you know the outcome. Not to succumb would be torment. One way to beat the cravings is to put as much distance as possible between you and the food. In other words, don't buy it.

Secondly, remember that cravings go. It is impossible to sustain desire, as anybody who has given up cigarettes will tell you. I gave up cigarettes. At first, you have to learn a completely new agenda for what to do in the times when you used to have a cigarette. You have to think yourself into a whole new person. What do non-smokers do? But after a few months things are not so bad and after a year you don't crave cigarettes at all. After ten years, I can tell you, you don't even think about them. Surely if you were hooked on cigarettes, it was impossible to do without them. Obviously not.

The same applies to food cravings. You cannot go without food, but you can give up things that are bad for you. Beating cravings means giving up completely, at least until you've got that habit or that food out of your system. That is why I never allow junk food or sweets on any of my diets. It is like offering an alcoholic a drink as a treat. You just wouldn't do it.

The 5-Day program banishes bad foods, but the Maintenance program does too. I'm not going to pretend that there is some weird and wonderful method for dealing with cravings. Why make life difficult for yourself by keeping the objects of your temptation around to torture you? You have to be strict, give them up and never look back. This is for your own good!

Allowing some "unlimited" foods

This is another tricky area. People always want to find some food in a diet that is "unlimited." This is to say that if you want more to eat, there is some food with which you can pile your plate as high as you like. Well, I am afraid I call this gluttony. If you are serious about learning new eating habits, unlimited food has to go. Even nibbling on raw carrots. If you have a problem with food, you must learn to eat smaller portions. On my diet, nothing is unlimited.

This is not to say that I blame you. I was taught to eat everything on the plate. We had healthy eating habits, but my mother could whip up her special rich dessert in no time, and we were encouraged to eat as much of it as possible. I never put on what we called weight in those days, because the culture was that if you gained a few pounds, you made sure you lost them pretty fast. However, controlling my gargantuan appetite was a challenge and I managed it by pretending to be a film star who toyed with tiny, stylish portions. This trick works.

If you have a big appetite and don't have a weight problem, you can have any unlimited food you like. But if you are overweight and yearn for a flatter stomach, you have to meet me halfway and give up the nibbling. Don't have unlimited amounts of food. Think stylish, and get your appetite down.

3 You Are Constipated

If there is anything worse than food going through you too quickly, it is food going through too slowly! You feel full and you look it. Constipation can be caused by:

- eating too much meat
- eating a high protein diet generally
- drinking too much tea
- eating too little fiber
- not drinking enough water
- some iron tablets
- some anti-depressant drugs.

Long-term use of laxatives can be extremely harmful to your body, as they prevent it from functioning in its own natural way and the end result is a lazy gut. They also cause a lot of fluid to be lost from the body, which you aren't aware of until you have a blinding headache.

People used to shovel down massive quantities of fiber because they believed it was healthy. It is, but it is also irritating to the stomach and this is what it is meant to be. Dealing with constipation – and I am all too aware that this is hardly an elegant topic – is easily done on your 5-Day program by having what is in effect a laxative evening meal or supper. All those vegetables which you couldn't eat during the day, like corn and fava beans, can now be eaten with abandon, and my recommended nightly dessert of fruit and yogurt is a treat you have to look forward to!

The last two causes of a big stomach, poorly toned muscles and bad posture, are dealt with in the section "Exercise and Posture."

A Quick Guide to Nutrition

A common misconception is that if you want a healthy, nutritious diet, you have to spend a fortune on fancy, gourmet foods. In fact, as long as you satisfy your body's needs for the right balance of carbohydrates, proteins and fats, you needn't spend more than a few dollars a week, a lot less than you would if you constantly snacked on chocolate and ate takeout.

My diet is particularly satisfying because there are no long periods without food. It does not have a huge amount of bulk, but it is quite high in carbohydrates – the foods that supply ready energy.

Carbohydrates

If you are stuck for a definition of a carbohydrate, think of anything that was a leaf, root, fruit, seed, nut, or grain. Plants, in other words. Even a simple spinach leaf has carbohydrates in it.

Carbohydrates fall into two categories: simple and complex.

They come in three main forms: sugars, starch and fiber.

Simple carbohydrates are sugars:

■ lactose is found in milk and dairy products and is half as sweet as sugar
■ glucose is found in vegetables, fruit and honey
■ sucrose is found in fruit and vegetables
■ fructose is found in fruit and honey
■ maltose is found in malt extract, barley, grains and malted wheat.

Complex carbohydrates include starches found in bread, potatoes, rice, pasta, cereals and nuts, as well as fibers found in unrefined foods.

Most carbohydrates are broken down during digestion. Although insoluble fiber is not digested, it nourishes bacteria in the large bowel and there is subsequent fermentation – need I say more?

However, do not exclude fiber for good. There is another type of fiber called soluble fiber, which is more easily absorbed by the gut and which is found in the following foods:

■ Quaker oats
■ fruit
■ vegetables.

Soluble fiber has many health benefits and is included in your 5-Day program. It helps reduce cholesterol in the blood and also slows the absorption of glucose, preventing sudden rises in blood sugar – particularly useful for diabetics.

Be wary of resistant starch. This is a type of starch that cannot be broken down by enzymes in the small intestine in the normal way. It is found in raw potatoes, unripe fruit, and some processed foods. It passes undigested into the large intestine where it can ferment, causing flatulence and extreme discomfort. You have been warned!

A high-carbohydrate diet replenishes and increases the body's reserves of glycogens, which play an important role in providing a readily usable energy supply and making you feel lively. A common complaint of dieters over the years has been the tiredness that almost inevitably accompanies low-calorie diets, but by eating the correct balance of proteins, carbohydrates and fats you should be able to lose weight steadily, and with no ill effects.

Proteins

Although only about twenty percent of our daily nutritional requirements are for protein, every cell in the human body needs it. Without it, tissue cannot be repaired effectively, nor can new cells grow. If you starve yourself on diets that give you hardly anything to eat, you are also doing a disservice to your looks. Proteins such as keratin and collagen keep your skin supple and young-looking and your hair strong and elastic. Protein also helps fight infection and aids digestion.

You will be nourished by a good balance of proteins on this diet.

Proteins come from two sources: plants and animals.

- **Animal proteins** cheese, fish, meat, poultry, millk, and eggs
- **Plant proteins** wheat, beans, bread, potatoes, rice, and nuts

Proteins cannot be stored by the body. Excess proteins are converted to glucose by the liver. If your diet is too rich in protein – for example, if you eat a lot of cheese or meat, you run the risk of osteoporosis because, strange as it may seem when you are eating calcium from cheese, too much protein can result in loss of calcium.

On the 5-Day program you will be eating most of the proteins listed above, with the exception of beans, and with only a very small amount of nuts, of which you need only a small quantity anyway. Just two Brazil nuts every day provide the average body with all it needs of some minerals, such as selenium, and also provide useful amounts of fat. A simple bowl of cereal with milk provides roughly one third of our daily recommended protein intake, so it is unlikely that many of us are deficient in protein.

Fats

Fat is essential. Without it, vitamins A, D and E cannot be absorbed from the gut and you can become severely vitamin-deficient, leading to illness. Fats form every membrane in every cell of the human body. It is vital that you do not exclude fat from your everyday meals.

Like proteins, fats also come from two sources: plant and animal. The "fat issue" is often a source of worry and topic of conversation, and ignorance is usually the cause. So here is a simple breakdown of the types of fat in our foods.

Animal fats

These are the so-called bad fats, found in:
- dairy foods
- milk
- meat.

In fact, all these foods were also in our list of proteins. The saturated fat (see below) contained in these foods is considered to be bad for the health of your heart. A rule of thumb is that if the fat is the type that solidifies when cooled after heating (like lard), it is less good for you.

Vegetable fats

Vegetable fats are mainly oils like olive oil, sunflower oil and oil from nuts which contain a high proportion of unsaturated fatty acids (see below). They are generally thought to be better for health, although this is irrelevant when considering the question of weight loss, as all fats contain the same number of calories per ounce.

Saturated and unsaturated

Fats are made up of fatty acids. The two main types of fats are saturated and unsaturated. Saturated fats are solid at room temperature – like butter – and are found in most animal products, such as eggs, milk and meat. Unsaturated fats are liquid, like sunflower oil. The unsaturated fats are then divided into monounsaturated and polyunsaturated. Saturated and monounsaturated fatty acids can be manufactured by the body from carbohydrates, alcohol and protein, so it is not essential to take extra supplies. Sources of monounsaturated fats include avocados, nuts, seeds, olive oil and fish oils.

Some polyunsaturated fatty acids cannot be made by the body and must therefore be taken in the form of the foods which contain them. These fatty acids are therefore called "essential," and are made up of two groups called Omega-6 (found in vegetable oils) and Omega-3 (found in soy bean oil, rapeseed oil, oily fish, such as sardines, herrings, mackerel and salmon and the liver of white fish).

An adult requires about 4g of Omega-6 fatty acids a day (a handful of almonds or two teaspoons of sunflower oil) with a maximum of 25g. Very high intakes may be harmful. Omega-3 fatty acids are needed in small amounts: 1–2g a day (a handful of walnuts or a small portion of oily fish). Deficiency in either fatty acid can lead to poor growth, skin problems and a weakened immune system.

Transfats

Transfats are added to products to prevent them becoming hard and rancid. Look out for "hydrogenated" on labels of foods such as margarine. They are found mainly in processed foods, such as chips, cakes and cookies.

On this diet you will not need to concern yourself with transfats as you won't be eating processed foods.

Fat is a necessary part of any good diet, but the key to healthy eating and weight loss is the percentage of your daily diet which fats make up. Experts disagree, but a sensible level would be no more than twenty percent of your diet.

Vitamins and Minerals

Each individual will have different nutritional needs, but it is fair to say that guidelines can be set for the average man or woman who is in good health, regardless of occupation, age, or size. The only adjustments which need to be taken into account are for very old people and young children, for pregnant and/or nursing mothers, and for people engaged in particularly strenuous physical activity.

Vitamins are usually classed as water-soluble or fat-soluble. Water-soluble vitamins are all the B vitamins and vitamin C, and they cannot be stored by the body as any excess is excreted in the urine. Thus, a person who takes a massive amount of vitamin C each day in the hope that it will be stored to ward off a cold is wasting money. Never take too many vitamins, as they can be poisonous to the system. Always read the label on the bottle.

Vitamins A, D, E and K are fat-soluble, which means that they need an intake of fat to be absorbed. Unlike water-soluble vitamins, these are stored by the body which means that any excess can be extremely dangerous for your health.

Essential minerals

A balanced diet will also include adequate amounts of some trace elements and minerals, including calcium and iron, and it is important to know their sources.

Iron – sources include red meat, legumes, oatmeal, wholegrain bread, nuts, parsley, egg yolks and fortified breakfast cereals. Iron is lost through perspiration, so supplements might be needed if you exercise a lot.

Calcium – sources include milk and butter, cheese, nuts, sunflower seeds, soy products and leafy vegetables.

Folic acid – sources include leafy vegetables, beans, eggs, peanuts, fruit and wholegrain cereals.

Vegetarians and vegans, in particular, have need of non-meat sources of iron and vitamin B12.

Other minerals such as iodine and manganese, known as trace elements, are needed in tiny amounts, while potassium, sodium and magnesium are needed in quite large quantities. However, on this diet, you will be eating all you require of these minerals.

Vitamin supplements

Should you be taking vitamin or mineral supplements on this diet? Many people pop dozens of pills every day without the slightest idea of what they are taking or whether they need them. I don't take any supplements at all. That is not to say that I recommend everyone to stay supplement-free, and if you are a pregnant or a nursing mother, have been ill, or are elderly it might be good to check with your doctor that you are 100 percent fit and healthy without supplements.

But do remember that supplements are exactly that. They are in addition to your food and not instead of it.

What most people don't realize, however, is that these nutrients are lost in different ways and at different rates according to our lifestyles, and no two people's needs are the same.

Stress and anxiety count for the loss of many nutrients from the body, as does an active lifestyle, so a very busy person could need extra vitamins and minerals. If you smoke, you lose 25mg (3/4oz) of vitamin C every time you light up. Cigarette smoking inhibits the absorption of vitamin C, as does the polluted atmosphere of an inner city, so if this is you, you'll need a supplement.

Coffee and tea drinking also inhibit absorption of vitamins, so if you drink a lot of these (more than four–six cups a day), either cut down, switch to the caffeine-free varieties or take extra vitamins. The small amount of vitamins you are losing may not seem much, but remember that the effect is cumulative. If you drink some caffeine, have the odd cigarette, drink alcohol daily, live in the city and have a pressured life, you are practically picking out tombstones! The point is, we can generally get away with it while we are young. We can smoke, drink, and party all night, and still bounce out of bed in the morning looking fabulous. Wait a few years, though, and you'll have a different tale to tell. I know of countless women who speak of their past excesses with regret. You don't want to live like a hermit, but neither do you want to end up in a few years' time with a bad back and looking like a raddled old bag, all because you couldn't be bothered to take a bit of care.

It goes without saying that an active lifestyle demands more from your body. Keen exercisers need extra iron, as they lose iron through sweating, and of course strict slimmers should take a multivitamin and mineral supplement every day – or maybe not be such strict slimmers.

If you drink alcohol heavily, not only are you damaging your health through dehydration and liver toxicity, but you could be in danger of a deficiency of thiamine (vitamin B1) which is needed to convert carbohydrates and fats into energy. Symptoms include lethargy, muscle weakness and numbness.

As I have said, vitamin A in quantity can be toxic and extremely hazardous to health. Pregnant women should avoid eating liver for this reason, and should never take a vitamin A supplement due to possible damage to the unborn baby.

If you have been neglecting yourself, then this 5-Day plan will be a breath of fresh air. Because we all have different needs due to age and lifestyle, I suggest you get personalized advice on vitamin and mineral supplements. This program, however, gives you all the nutrients you need.

THE
Diet

So What Am I Going to Eat?

I bet you typically begin a diet taking off on a shopping spree at your local supermarket. Your kitchen usually looks like you're preparing for Thanksgiving as you fill your fridge with chicken breasts and salad greens, and load up on fruit. Surely this is the right way to go about a new, healthy regime, right?

Well, yes and no. It's a good idea to get rid of the junk food you've stocked up on and consider healthy substitutes, but perhaps filling your kitchen with various foods isn't the best idea. Maybe you should think this through a little more. Could it be that you have developed a preoccupation with food and that this is what got you into trouble in the first place?

Learning about tasty, inventive ways with food is wonderful if you have a settled relationship with food. It's fine to be a food-lover if you don't have a weight problem. But if you're reducing, it's not so good. Giving you a long grocery list is like giving an alcoholic a job as a bartender. Why torture you—and why should you torture yourself?

Save your gourmet recipes for the day you're slim. The Maintenance program allows more leeway so that you can indulge yourself on special occasions or when entertaining. When you've got your stomach deliciously flat you won't want to spoil it. Anyway, fancy recipes can lead to munching while you cook; even if it's only a vegetable, that old hand-to-mouth reflex will soon have you reaching for a doughnut. Train yourself out of it!

Meals on your 5-Day program are simple, delicious and most important, nutritious. You will be beautifying your body as well as giving it a break. I know you might have others to feed, but this way you can do your own thing during the day and join everybody else in the evening for a good meal.

And simple food doesn't have to be boring. If you love elegant meals, serve your chicken and spinach on your best china. Sit down as though you were dining out. Smoked salmon, herb omelettes, and shrimp salads can be fancy and gourmet. Small portions are chic. Remind yourself that plain food is fabulous for your figure. So prepare yourself and buckle down for the next few days, and get a week's supply of yogurt, fish, and oatmeal. Don't get more than you can eat in a week. And think thin. This is going to be a strict diet. You can do it.

The Rules—Start By Getting Strict

It is necessary that you take yourself in hand now, so keep to these golden rules.

DO

1 eat every three hours
2 drink water between meals
3 steer clear of starchy carbohydrates and high-fiber foods during the day
4 eat your fruit during the evening
5 stick to the portion-control rules—nothing is unlimited.

DO NOT

1 use artificial sweeteners
2 buy or eat any ready-meals or fast food
3 skip breakfast
4 go to bed hungry.

Your Guidelines for Eating

1 Do not put more on your plate than your portion allowances.
2 Try not to have second helpings.
3 Never load your fork or spoon with the next mouthful before you have swallowed the previous one.
4 If you feel full, stop eating. Put the plate aside and come back to it later.
5 Do not swallow your food until it is thoroughly chewed.
6 Where possible, as in the case of apples, slice food into manageable pieces rather than eat whole. Put on a plate and sit down to eat; this will encourage moderation.

I apologize if this sounds like a mother teaching her children table manners, but problems with food and weight often have their root cause in bad eating habits. Don't treat every meal as if you won't get the chance to eat ever again.

You do not have to go out and buy expensive foods like salmon and shrimp if you do not wish to. You might not have a kitchen which is equipped for a lot of preparation and cooking, or you might live on your own and find making a whole dish just too complicated or time-consuming. However, the diet lasts only five days and is intended to produce results, so it's worth going out to get the recommended foods.

I have included a vegetarian recipe section and most of the pasta dishes are suitable for vegetarians, but I generally find that most vegetarians are experts at adapting ideas for their own tastes. Many of the recipes and menu choices are for use on the Maintenance Program only, of course.

What Will I Drink?

Sorry to be a party pooper. No alcohol is allowed on the 5-Day plan, but it won't kill you. When you progress to the Maintenance Program, you can have a couple of glasses of wine a day, beer, or the odd glass of champagne, if you choose.

Try not to drink much water with your meal. It is fine to have a glass of water handy, especially when you are with others as they might think it odd if you do not drink at all, but take small sips. Add a slice of fresh lemon or maybe try orange to make it taste sweet and different. It is important not to drink massive quantities of water with food because your stomach acids need to be strong for good digestion. Weak digestive juices mean your food will not be digested as robustly and this can lead to indigestion and feeling that your meal "just hasn't gone down."

Have plenty of water between meals. Aim to drink 2 liters (8 glasses) every day. In addition, drink tea and decaffeinated coffee as you wish. No carbonated drinks are allowed. Remember that they encourage gas in the intestines which can result in flatulence.

What If I Get Hungry?

I'll let you into a secret. I often have all-day photo-shoots dressed in a leotard and tight leggings. I have to stay in this garb for up to six hours and naturally I get hungry. But what about the flat stomach? I am doing exercise shots after all and it wouldn't do to find it hard to hold myself in!

I simply get a large tub of yogurt (with live and active cultures) and keep it by the set. Every half hour or so I take another spoonful. It keeps me going brilliantly because it bathes the stomach so I don't feel hungry. And as you know by now, yogurt has carbohydrates which give me energy. It needs hardly any digesting, so it's like putting liquid into a food processor – no grinding or chopping. I keep my flat tummy and I end the day without one second of hunger.

Now, I am not suggesting that you live on yogurt. But you'll find ways of compromising and sometimes you need liquids rather than solids to keep grumbling at bay. Thirst can feel like hunger. Have a drink of water or nonfat milk but *always wait to eat until your next scheduled meal.* Picking at food and snacking are terrible for waking up a nicely snoozing tummy and setting all that grinding off again.

Nearly There . . .

Before you get going, you need to get rid of the past. You are entering a new phase of your life – the newer, better version of yourself. You bear a striking resemblance to the old you, but you are not the same person. Act as if you are taking over this person's house after she has moved out and start by chucking out all her old rubbish.

1 Give away all those packets of dried fruit and cans of baked beans that are sitting at the back of your pantry. Somebody will appreciate them.

2 Tell the family that you don't want bad food in the house. Insist they don't have it – you are in charge of what your children eat, after all. If you live with someone, you can still eat what they are having in the evening – just a bit less of it. This is not going to affect their meals at all.

3 Buy what you need – don't "stock up." This isn't a siege. Get a week's supply of foods like chicken, fish, avocados, fruits and vegetables, potatoes, pasta and rice. Buy plenty of yogurt that contains live and active cultures, cottage cheese, milk and oats.

4 Weigh yourself, take measurements and write them down here. I suggest:

Weight _____

Over bust under armpits _____

Bust line at fullest point _____

Under bust _____

Waist _____

Just below the navel _____

In line with the public bone _____

Hips at fullest point _____

Each thigh approximately six inches below top of legs

left _____ right_____

3 inches above each knee

left _____ right_____

Each calf

left _____ right_____

Each ankle

left _____ right_____

These measurements give you the best possible "snapshot" of your figure. If fat is lost from the back (and this is often the second place to go – the first is the face) your bust measurement will be smaller. If you lose weight from your buttocks, your abdominal measurement will go down. If you tone up your buttocks you might find your abdomen feels tight. In addition, you can often *feel* fat and be convinced you have gained weight, or feel thin and think you can relax, but the gentle reminder of these few statistics will tell another story. I still have the measurements I wrote down in my 1977 diary – so I know where the fat has gone! Since then I have taken my measurements every January, which, I can tell you, makes fascinating reading. So please make a note of your statistics as well as your weight – there will be no excuse for not knowing if you have made progress!

Basic Rules Before You Get Started

■ Eat breakfast within an hour of waking. If you are going to the gym or for a run, etc., and you won't be having breakfast until later, have a small snack like a few tablespoons of yogurt, a glass of milk, or two tablespoons of plain oats soaked in milk before you go.

■ Eat from a 9-inch dinner plate. Go and buy one if you don't have one already. This simply keeps portions small as you cannot actually pile more onto your plate. Do not have second helpings, either!

■ Eat sitting down, at a table. Never spend less than ten minutes, preferably fifteen to twenty minutes, eating any one course.

■ Measure portions by the tablespoon.

■ Ban all foods sweetened with sorbitol or aspartame.

■ Have plenty of water between meals: Aim to drink 2 liters (8 glasses) every day.

Recommended Foods

Plain yogurt, with live and active cultures

I cannot recommend yogurt highly enough. It is a complete food, meaning it contains all three main food groups: protein, carbohydrate and fat together. Few foods have them all. Your yogurt should contain mildly fermented "live" cultures of L-acidophilus, L. Casei and Bifidobacterium. Check the container for information.

3½oz (100g) plain yogurt has approximately 4.2g protein, 3.5g fat and 5.3g carbohydrates.

Plain oats

Oats contain soluble fiber, which is extra kind to your insides. The carbohydrates help keep you full for longer, and the steady release of energy ensures you feel good and beat tiredness slumps.

1oz (30g) oats has 3.7g protein, 2.6g fat and 22g carbohydrates.

Fish

You can eat any fish! Kind to the gut, you may pan-fry it in butter, poach it in milk, grill or steam it. Other ways with fish are given in the recipe section, but suffice to say that you won't be bored with your fish.

5oz (150g) white fish has about 26g protein, 4.8g fat and a trace of carbohydrate.

5oz (150g) oily fish, such as salmon or mackerel, has 24–34g protein, 13–28g fat and no carbohydrate, although it is important to note that the fat is mostly monounsaturated and therefore healthy, and the saturated fat content is as low as 2–5g.

A small can of tuna fish has around 25g protein, 8g fat and no carbohydrate.

3½oz (100g) shellfish, like shrimp and crab, have 14g protein, almost no fat at 0.5g and no carbohydrate.

Eggs

Eggs are wonderful. It is probably because I have chickens at home, but I have always based my diet on eggs – not surprising when I only have to walk down to the nest box and collect a handful of freshly laid, nutritious eggs. And they're such powerhouses of goodness! I routinely hard-boil half a dozen to keep ready in my fridge from where I can slice and scatter them over a salad, slice onto melba toast for a light meal, put into a sandwich or just eat whole.

A plate of scrambled or poached eggs or a three-egg omelette has 19g protein, 5.4g fat and no carbohydrates.

Leafy greens

You are avoiding sprouts, cabbage, etc., but should eat what I am calling "leafy greens." Basically, if it is a leaf, it is OK. These include spinach, lettuce, watercress and so on. You can also have chicory, peeled cucumber, zucchini and squash. If in doubt, ask yourself if your vegetable came from under or above the ground. I am not being too prescriptive in case your diet includes some greens I have never heard of, but it is safe to eat all leaves. Do not include roots at this point. Root vegetables are higher in carbohydrates and can cause a small but significant reaction in your system. By all means have them during the evening, but do not choose them for the daytime.

A standard portion of leafy greens has around 2g protein, a trace of fat and less than 1g of carbohydrates.

Chicory has somewhat more carbohydrates, but that is per head of chicory.

Summary of Important Permitted Foods

These foods can be eaten freely on your Maintenance Program, but bear in mind the guidance on portion control

Fish	Poultry	Meat	Dairy
salmon	skinned chicken	lamb	yogurt, with live and
tuna	skinned turkey	pork	active cultures
smoked haddock**	pheasant	beef*	nonfat milk
smoked salmon**	duck	venison	cottage cheese
white cod and haddock	goose	lean ham**	hard cheese
halibut	quail	lean bacon**	eggs
trout			
sardines			
shrimp/prawns			
scallops			
crab			
lobster			

*Beef is digested slowly and
  can cause constipation.
** High in sodium and
  preservatives. Eat sparingly.

Vegetables eat freely any time
romaine lettuce, watercress, arugula, peppers, field greens, radicchio, french or string beans, zucchini, avocado, chicory, spinach, beets, jicama

Fruits eat with care after 6 p.m.
grapes, apples, apricots, plums, baked fruits, blackcurrants, raspberries, mango, pineapple, strawberries, bananas, all dried fruit

Fats and dressings OK to eat in moderation
unsalted butter, fresh mayonnaise, half and half or pouring cream, olive oil, sunflower oil, walnut oil, sesame oil

Cereals during the day eat these only
Quaker oats, Rice Krispies, Special K

Nuts eat after 6 p.m. only
Brazil nuts, hazelnuts, almonds, unsalted cashew nuts, walnuts, sunflower seeds, pine nuts

Grains eat after 6 p.m. only, or avoid altogether
Shredded Wheat, rice, pasta, bran flakes, All-Bran

Vegetables eat after 6 p.m. only
carrots, parsnips, potatoes, tomatoes, sweetcorn, peas, fava beans

Exclude Completely

Vegetables

- mushrooms
- baked beans
- lima beans
- kidney beans
- onions
- chickpeas

Fats

- low-fat spreads – *do not eat*
- salted butter
- lard
- mayonnaise with emulsifiers and additives

Miscellaneous

- *all* cookies
- cakes
- muffins
- bagels
- baguettes
- sweets
- fruit yogurts
- very low-fat or low-calorie yogurts
- premade sandwiches
- "fast" food
- breadcrumbed products
- salted peanuts

Yeast-forming Foods

The following foods have a tendency to cause bloating. They are known as yeast-forming foods because they are held responsible for intestinal chaos that is sometimes a result of lingering bacterial infections, courses of antibiotics and taking the Pill or HRT treatment:

- peanuts
- pickles
- soy sauce
- ketchup
- vinegar
- grapes and wine
- beer and lager
- dried fruits
- ice cream
- gravy mixes
- sweet potatoes
- mushrooms.

It is by no means inevitable that you are sensitive to these foods, but it will not hurt to leave them out altogether during your initial five days. No worries, though, because there is plenty left to eat!

Cheese is included in the standard 5-Day program, but do see how you get on with it as some people find it tricky. Cottage cheese is fine, but I suggest you steer clear of blue-veined cheeses.

Portion Control

Portion size is big news. Sizes have doubled and even quadrupled in the past twenty years. Burgers are three times the size they used to be. Even food outlets that have salad bars allow "main meal" salads where you can pile your plate as high as you like and a whole generation is growing up with the notion that a twelve-inch (30cm) platter topped with an eight-ounce (225g) chicken breast, six roast potatoes, four tablespoons of each vegetable, and a mound of stuffing is a standard meal.

I am afraid it is not. People constantly write to me in amazement at their weight gain and protruding stomach and tell me they are eating exactly the same as they ate ten years ago. They aren't.

They might be eating the same food, but they are almost certainly eating at least thirty percent more of it.

If you are going to conquer your body, you need to conquer portions. The good news is that this is not going to mean a huge sacrifice. You will know by now that I hate substitute food and love the real thing. You might be shifting your meals around on the 5-Day program but you are not sacrificing much. Rather than give up chicken in cream sauce, you will have a smaller portion. And with time, you will wonder how you ever managed to eat so much.

Here Are Your Portion Sizes:

Vegetables

greens, carrots, etc. . . . . 2 tablespoons

peas, fava beans . . . . 2 tablespoons

mashed carrots . . . . 2 tablespoons

boiled or roast potatoes . . . . 2 small potatoes
or 3½ oz (100g)

mashed potato with skimmed
milk and 1 tsp of butter . . . . 2 tablespoons
or one scoop

baked potato. 5oz (150g)

Legumes

lentils. . . . . 2 tablespoons

Salads

Your salad plate should be no bigger than 7 inches (18cm).

field greens . . . . 4–6 leaves

cucumber. . . . . 4 slices

peppers . . . . 2–3 rings of each

sweetcorn. . . . . 1 tablespoon

grated carrot. . . . . 1 tablespoon

radishes . . . . 1 tablespoon

all other salad additions . . . keep portions small

Other

chicken, beef steak, lamb or
pork chop. 5oz (150g)

roasted meat . . . . 3 slices

casseroles. . . . . 2 tablespoons

pasta or rice . . . . 1/4 cup dry weight

bread . . . . 1 medium slice

rice pudding and other puddings . . 3 tablespoons

fruit compote . . . . 2–3 tablespoons

fish standard filet 4–6oz

butter. . . . . 4 tablespoons for 5 days

milk . . . . as much as you need

THE
5-Day
Diet

This plan should be followed for five days.

It is important that you keep to the plan and do not find reasons why it will not work for you, for example not liking yogurt or oats is a poor excuse to not follow this program. This is like asking your doctor for different medication when he gives you the best cure for your problem.

This diet offers my best advice and when followed exactly, it entirely works. If you decide to change it, I cannot guarantee the outcome.

The simplicity of the 5-Day program not only helps you lose weight and reduce bloating, but it frees you from the stress of endless choices. However, if you want more variety, you can find suggestions for alternative meals on page 48.

To the best of my ability, I have worked with standard working hours and patterns. I know you might have a different schedule, in which case observe the basic rules: no high-fiber fruits, vegetables, or grains when you are active or during the day.

Forget any fancy notions of "no carbs after 6pm." If you're a night owl and work late, it could be six hours between dinner and bedtime. That's when you need your late night snack, especially the milk and honey. It will tide over your blood sugar levels until morning and guarantee a good night's sleep.

Advance Preparation

Everybody is busy, so anything which you can prepare in advance helps you stay away from temptation in the kitchen.

Here are some suggestions:

1 When possible, try to make or cook two or more of foods like poached salmon and grilled chicken breast, which are both nice to have cold in salads. You then have a portion ready for the next day. Batch-cooking is a sensible idea that has kept me going on my busy schedule for years.
2 Always have hard-boiled eggs and grated cheese handy in the fridge.
3 Weigh out your ration of butter and put it in a separate dish in the fridge ready for use. This is 2oz (60g) for five days, or 3oz (85g) for a week.

Tip

Puréed, mashed or poached fruits and vegetables are a good shortcut to easing discomfort, bloating and flatulence. Sometimes you only need to remove the peel or skin, but I have always found that well-puréed carrot, parsnip and even broccoli—as if you were making it for a baby—can reduce the flatulence factor. I discovered this years ago when making meals for my children. After the inevitable "clearing up" of their leftovers, I didn't have any bloating! Some people yearn to have vegetables and fruit in their diet, but the tiniest spoonful blows them up, so either baby food or mashed/puréed fruit and vegetables are a good alternative. See if it works for you, because it is not guaranteed. *Experiment!*

day 1

* Asterisk indicates recipe included in back of book

Breakfast
Oatmeal (1/4 cup of oats and water) served with nonfat millk and honey, if desired
OR
Oatmeal soaked overnight in nonfat milk, topped with
1 tsp yogurt and a drizzle of honey

Mid-morning
Small serving (6 oz) yogurt
OR
Small cup coffee with nonfat milk, 1 tsp sugar if desired

Lunch
3 slices cold turkey, chicken or beef (about 4–6ozs) with
mixed green salad and 1 tbsp vinaigrette

Mid-afternoon
Small serving (6oz) yogurt
OR
Small cup coffee with nonfat milk, no sugar

Dinner
Grilled or pan-fried salmon fillet
(cook one extra and refrigerate for tomorrow)
WITH
Peas and mixed green salad
AND
Medium baked potato with 2 tsps sour cream
OR
Pasta Primavera* and mixed green side salad

Dessert
Small bowl of fiber-rich fruit salad (sliced strawberries, 1 sliced peach,
6 halved grapes and half a grated apple)
Serve with 1 tsp sour cream

Late Evening (if hungry)
1 apple, 1 banana, 6 almonds or Brazil nuts
Small cup warm nonfat milk with 1 tsp honey

day 2

Breakfast
Oatmeal ($1/4$ cup oats and water) served with nonfat milk and honey, if desired
OR
2 scrambled or poached eggs, 2 slices of lean bacon
(Grill extra bacon and leave cold, break into small pieces and save)

Mid-morning
Small cup of coffee with nonfat milk, no sugar
OR
Regular glass (10oz) nonfat milk with honey

Lunch
Cold salmon or tuna from last night's dinner
WITH
Mixed green salad, tomatoes and shredded carrots, oil and vinaigrette
OR
Cottage cheese (10oz) with mixed green salad

Mid-afternoon
Small serving (6 oz) live and active cultures yogurt
OR
Bowl of mixed green salad with vinaigrette

Dinner
Plain skinless, boneless turkey or chicken breast, grilled or roasted
(Cook two and have one cold tomorrow)
WITH
Julienne carrots, broccoli
4 small boiled new potatoes or 1 small baked potato (4oz), 1 tsp sour cream

Dessert
Grapes with sour cream and brown sugar*

Late Evening (if hungry)
1 apple, 1 banana, 6 almonds or Brazil nuts
Small cup warm nonfat milk, with 1 tsp honey

day 3

Breakfast

Oatmeal (¼ cup oats and water) served with nonfat milk and honey, if desired
OR
¼ cup Rice Krispies, no sugar, teacup nonfat milk

Mid-morning

Small serving (6 oz) yogurt
OR
Small cup coffee with nonfat milk, 1 tsp sugar if desired

Lunch

Herb Omelette Salad*
OR
Cold chicken breast mixed with bacon pieces from yesterday
Bind with 2 tsp sour cream or mayonnaise
Serve with mixed green salad

Mid-afternoon

Bowl of mixed green salad with vinaigrette
OR
Glass (10oz) nonfat milk with honey

Dinner

Skinny chicken and garden grill*
OR
Salmon with almond and honey crust with mashed potatoes (6 oz)
(mashed with nonfat milk, no butter)
2 or 3 green vegetables, steamed

Dessert

6 plums (fresh or canned) served with rice pudding (3 tbsp)
3 pineapple slices, roasted, served with 1 tsp tsp lowfat sour cream

Late Evening (if hungry)

1 apple, 1 banana, 6 almonds or Brazil nuts
Small cup warm nonfat milk with 1 tsp honey

day 4

Breakfast
Oatmeal (¼ cup oats and water) served with nonfat milk and honey, if desired
OR
Omelette made from 2 whole eggs and two egg whites,
Filled with 1 tbsp cottage cheese

Mid-morning
Small serving (6oz) yogurt
OR
Glass (10oz) nonfat milk with honey

Lunch
Caesar salad*
OR
Salade Nicoise*

Mid-afternoon
Half an avocado
OR
Small cup coffee with nonfat milk, no sugar

Dinner
Shrimp Portofino*
OR
Beef in Red Wine*
WITH
Mashed potatoes, spinach and carrots

Dessert
Fiber-rich fruit salad (sliced strawberries, 1 sliced peach,
6 halved grapes and half a grated apple)
Served with 1tsp sour cream

Late Evening (if hungry)
1 apple, 1 banana, 6 almonds or Brazil nuts
Small cup warm nonfat milk with1 tsp honey

day 5

Breakfast
Oatmeal (¼ cup oats and water) served with nonfat milk and honey, if desired
OR
Oatmeal soaked in milk, with 1 tsp of yogurt and drizzle of honey

Mid-morning
Mixed green salad with small handful of parmesan shavings,
vinaigrette with added juice of one orange
OR
Small serving (6oz) yogurt

Lunch
Smoked salmon (4oz), 1 tsp sour cream, capers and half an avocado,
sliced, served on mixed green salad, with lemon to squeeze over
OR
½ cup of cottage cheese with vegetable sticks (celery, carrots, peppers)

Mid-afternoon
Small serving yogurt
OR
Small cup coffee with nonfat milk, no sugar

Dinner
Cheese omelette with grated carrot, spinach and sweetcorn
Small baked potato (4oz)
OR
Home-made grilled or barbecued hamburgers*
With dry-roast oven chips* (6oz)
and 1 tbsp Fiery Sundried Tomato Salsa*

Dessert
3 pineapple slices, roasted, served with 1 tsp sour cream

Late Evening (if hungry)
1 apple, 1 banana, 6 almonds or Brazil nuts
Small cup warm nonfat milk with 1 tsp honey

More Meal Choices

I have made your daily menus pretty rigid for the five days. Experience tells me that people prefer everything to be set down for them to follow. Sometimes, though, you need to be a little more flexible, so here are some other main meal ideas.

These are not to be eaten during the day. Keep them for after 6 p.m., when they can do less damage. I have not given recipes for all these meals as some will be familiar dishes you will be able to make without detailed instructions.

Mediterranean Cod
Salade Nicoise
Salmon with Almond and Honey Crust
Crab and Rice Ball Salad
Scallop and Bacon Provencale
Smoked Salmon Potato Cakes with Dill Cream
Grilled Chicken in Orange Marinade
Chicken with Almonds
Skinny Chicken and Garden Grill
Chicken with Watermelon and Hazelnut Salad
Moroccan Chicken Salad
Lemon Paprika Chicken with Walnuts and Bowtie Pasta
Greek Chicken Salad
Caeser Salad (V)
Wild Rice and Pecan Salad (V)
Cannelloni Stuffed with Spinach and Almonds (V)
Herb, Cheese or Spanish Omelette (V)
Baked Cheese Tomatoes (V)
Vinaigrette
Homemade Fiery Sundried Tomato Salsa
Grapes with Sour Cream and Brown Sugar
Rice Pudding

Exercise
AND
Posture

Doing It the Natural Way

If you want to succeed with your fabulously flat stomach, you have to get moving. These days "exercise" has come to mean something rather formal at the gym, but the difference between exercise and movement is like the difference between taking your dog for a walk on a leash, and simply opening the door to let it wander around the garden. Both would have the same result. In the same way, all types of movement count as exercise and if you are relying on daily sit-ups to flatten that tummy for you, you might have to wait a rather long time.

Put it like this: there are twenty-four hours in a day and if you only tone your abs for fifteen minutes a day, that leaves a lot of time for them to get out of shape! The great thing about natural movement is (a) you don't realize you are doing it, (b) it's instant and free, (c) it gets better results because your muscles are being toned all the time. The 5-Day program relies on natural effort, a healthy lifestyle and the great outdoors. You can walk anywhere at any time. Go out to post a letter, rather than saving it for when you drive by the box. Cancel the newspaper delivery and walk or jog to the shop instead. If you are concerned about safety, go mall-walking; that's walking around your local shopping center where you have stairs, a climate-controlled environment and restrooms!

I am very much an outdoors person and urge you to try it for yourself. It is so great for your figure and you get several jobs done at once – gardening or shopping or whatever plus a wonderful flat stomach.

Completing the Circle

Working on your abs to the exclusion of everything else will only do a third of the job. The whole abdominal section of your body is what I call your "midcircle" and you must exercise the whole of it.

You will target:

■ your oblique muscles (the ones that run down the side of your trunk)

■ your rectus abdominis muscle (the one that if overdeveloped forms the "six-pack" appearance)

■ your hip flexors (they start at your hips and run down your legs and can help to tone your lower abdominal area)

■ your back muscles – to help you stand up straight without thinking about it.

In order of effectiveness, here are my top exercises for the midcircle:

1 Swimming
This tones all your muscles, moves joints in their full range, stretches and tones your abdominals and obliques and strengthens your back.

2 Sweeping, raking, vacuuming
Really hard sweeping or raking is good for your abdominals as long as you remember to pull in your tummy before you start. Thereafter, each sweeping move towards you contracts your abdominals.

3 Washing the floor
I don't know if you have ever seen or used an ab-roller, but washing a floor on hands and knees is the same movement that you would get using one of those toning gadgets. You need to be on your knees, reaching out with one arm and then the other, or both together. The act of reaching and then drawing your arms towards you on the floor is fabulous for toning your abs. Five minutes is enough.

Which Exercise?

It is always assumed that if people simply exercise more, then their figure problems will disappear. If only. Cycling will not improve your abdominals, neither will step aerobics. You need the right exercise for your own needs and, right now, we want a flatter stomach.

If you are a complete beginner, if you have health problems, bad knees and have never walked further than the kitchen, you won't want to start with 100 sit-ups before breakfast. But neither will you welcome my suggestion of a gentle morning stroll if you've just completed the New York Marathon. The main thing to do, though, is to increase whatever you are doing now, and to do more floor exercises every day. So if you are doing nothing in the way of exercise, it's best to start with about five minutes of warm-up and stomach-tightening exercises, adding some aerobic exercise every day. If you are a hot-shot expert, go with advanced abdominal exercises five times a day, and an extra forty-five minutes of aerobic work such as swimming or cycling. Whatever you are doing, do more of it!

Muscle Toning – What Is It?

Every muscle is toned simply by being moved. Toning just means it is doing something. People will often "tone" themselves with weights, but weights build muscle, adding to their size and capability. When you do your midcircle exercises, I want you to tone your muscles, not build them. Building them will result in bigger muscles and you could even find your waist thickening and your abdomen bulging.

This is not as crazy as it sounds. A friend of mine went from flab to fab eight years ago, but got hooked on her ever flatter tummy. Soon she was adding weights to her sit-up routines and doing those exercises where you hang by your knees from a bar and sit up – holding twenty-pound (9kg) weights! Needless to say, she had an impressive six-pack. Today, that six-pack has turned into a fat-free but loose set of muscles, hanging limp as a spare tire under her T-shirt. Not a good look. On this plan, you will be toning your muscles with your own bodyweight.

Stretch Bands

You can't look good if you don't stretch. Modern ways of exercising have left women with bowed, muscular thighs, thick ankles, and large calves. Many women would call themselves fit, yet they can't straighten their knees. Nor can they press a hand into the space between their shoulder blades or touch their toes. They might have a body–fat ratio to die for, but total fitness includes having muscles that can operate over a large range, and that means they should be flexible and easily stretched to avoid injury. An individual who is fit but not flexible cannot be said to have all-round fitness.

Beauty is an entire effect. Some people train themselves into the ground for their beautiful body and then shower and slouch off with their sports bag weighing down their shoulders. No thought of elegance. No line to the body or beauty of movement. No point.

Flexibility training should be included as part of your daily activities from now on and that is why I recommend stretch bands (also known as flex or Pilates bands). They are a specific resistance and length and are your ultimate tool for stretching, lengthening and toning that midcircle – and all in one tiny band that you can pack in your luggage when you travel. A flat stomach depends on having a nice line to your body with long, lean and stretched muscles. With stretch bands you lengthen your abdominals and waist and can improve the appearance of your stomach by several inches.

Now, you do not have to use a stretch band. If you are elderly, not physically strong because you have been ill, or simply do not wish to have a band, then you don't have to use one. Your normal abdominal exercises from the next section will be quite enough to flatten your abs and give you noticeably toned muscles.

However, there is no substitute for the band, as it is immensely strong and will not snap, allowing extremes of safe movement.

A Quick Calorie Count

I don't approve of counting calories for the sake of it, but just for fun, and to cheer you up if you are stuck in an office or at home and can't get out much, here is a list of the calories spent doing a variety of ordinary chores:

Calories per half-hour:

Sleeping 30

Sweeping 90

Making beds 120

Typing 60

Standing still 45

Driving 60

Eating 45

Mowing the lawn 225

Washing dishes 60

Digging the garden 240

Washing clothes 90

Moderate cycling 120

Writing 60

Racing cycling 330

Ironing 60

Knitting 45

Aerobics 200–300

Mopping the floor 120

Brisk walking 180

Exercising at Home

I admit that I am quite vain. I was conscious of wanting a good figure even when my children were small. With limited time and absolutely no facilities or babysitters, I did what everybody did – got down on the floor for five precious minutes when the children were napping and did my stretch and sit-up routine.

The 5-Day program was born from those days. This is a plan that works because it is about consistency rather than an unsustainable effort every six months. Think of it like a fantastic haircut. If you had a killer cut and expensive restyle would you expect it to look just as good after three months? Of course not. Would you blame the hairdresser and say the hairstyle "didn't work" if it was a total mess after a few weeks? You'd be mad to. But people say this all the time about diet and exercise plans which they have tried for a couple of months and then given up on. They say it didn't work.

Don't save all your exercise for the gym. Exercising at home is sensible body-maintenance which you have to do.

Here is your exercise program:

Always warm up
The purpose of a warm-up is to prepare the body for exercise. Muscles which are cold – and remember that even on the hottest day your muscles will not be ready for action if they have been at rest – will not stretch, and will tear easily.

Your Five Abdominal Exercises

I am going to give you just five variations on the standard stomach-strengthening exercise. They are:

1 the Foundation
2 the Crunch
3 the Waist Whittler
4 the Chair Lift
5 the Air Bike.

You do not have to do all the variations.

If you are new to abdominal exercise, if you have been ill or have had a baby, it is best to stay with the Foundation exercise until you are stronger. It will be quite enough to keep you toned and trim, and as you progress you can add in the Waist Whittler, which is another quite basic exercise. If you are already accustomed to exercise, I suggest you do all five exercises twice a day on alternate days.

Abdominal exercises are not always easy to get right. People complain that their neck aches and back hurts. If anything ever hurts, stop immediately. There can be several reasons for the pain:

1 Your position is wrong.
2 You have done too many repetitions.
3 You are tired.
4 It is the wrong time of the month.

This last reason is important because your monthly cycle can affect the way you exercise to quite a marked degree. In the week or so before your period, hormones are pouring into your body that mimic pregnancy in a small way, and your ligaments can be a little vulnerable. Around this time, women can suffer from minor injuries more easily than at other times, so take care.

The Foundation

1 Start off lying down with your feet flat on the floor, about hip-width apart.
2 Place both hands under the bulge at the back of your head. Look at the ceiling.
3 Lift your head, but let your hands take its weight.
4 Make your chest and your head and neck one piece, in one line. The best way to think of your upper position is that the line of your top half should not be broken by the hinge of the neck.
5 Inhale before you start. Exhale, as you press your stomach downwards towards the floor. Tilt your pelvis up towards your chest and neck. Lift your head without breaking the line by tugging on your head or jerking it upwards. Keep pressing your stomach down.

   This pattern of breathing should continue throughout. Breathe in before you start, or on the release of effort. Breathe out and press downwards at the point of maximum effort, i.e. when you lift. Breathe in as you slowly and gently lower your head back down towards the floor.

6 Good! Now you have mastered the form of the sit-up, do eight more repetitions.
7 Have a rest for ten seconds; bring your knees into your chest.
8 Repeat the exercise, doing eight or sixteen repetitions, according to how you feel.
9 Stretch out by turning over and lifting yourself on to your elbows. Remember to keep your head and neck in alignment with your spine by looking down at the floor while you do this.

The Crunch

1 This time, lie on the floor with your feet lifted off the floor and cross your ankles. Feel the small of your back pressed firmly to the floor.

2 Take your upper position, as for the Foundation, neck and chest in one line. Support your head with your hands. As before, do not pull on your neck. Your head and back should be in one line.

3 Breathe in, lift your chest and press your stomach downwards, exhaling as you do so. Lift and lower your head as in the Foundation four times, up and down, slowly, then do eight double-time pulses, then repeat the four slow crunches.

4 Turn over and stretch out as before to decompress your spine.

The Chair Lift

This exercise is slightly easier than the Crunch if you find it hard to keep your legs up. It also stops your legs from helping you, thereby giving your stomach muscles all the hard work!

1 Lie on the floor with your bottom about 18 inches from the base of a chair. Place your legs from the knee downwards on the chair. Put your hands under your head as in the previous exercises.
2 Breathe in to prepare. Breathe out, and press downwards with your abdomen, raising your upper body as you do so. You won't come up very high.
3 Lower as you breathe in, expanding your chest as you do so. Repeat eight times, rest and repeat a further eight.
4 Turn over and decompress your spine as before.
5 Return to your starting position and repeat the two sets of eight. Decompress.

The Air Bike

Only do this exercise if you are not severely over-weight, and if you can be sure to keep your legs up in the air. It isn't a failing if you find it hard – you'll work up to it soon enough!

1 Take position as in picture.
2 Pulse slowly up to each knee with the opposite elbow as it comes in towards your face, then stretch the leg out towards the ceiling. Do eight or sixteen slowly, depending on your level of fitness and strength.
3 Rest, repeat the set then turn over to stretch out, decompressing as before.

Do not swivel your elbows wildly from side to side

The Waist Whittler

Without exercise, your oblique muscles, which lie around your ribcage area and which shape your waist, sit there, do nothing and are slack. This exercise does not increase the number of muscle fibers because you are not using weight. It tones and stretches the muscles so they become taut, and give you a tighter, smaller waist.

1 Lie on your back, arms outstretched. Lift your feet off the floor, as shown, knees bent. Press your spine hard to the floor and breathe in.

2 Now breathe out as you allow your legs to roll to one side, slowly. Keep your legs touching all the time. Stop short of the floor or go as far as you can. Hold and breathe in again, tightening your abdominal muscles and checking the position of your shoulders, which should still be on the floor.

3 Breathe out and, using your torso muscles, bring your legs back to center and then over to the opposite side. Repeat this move slowly, about three times to each side. If you can do more, great. But you must keep both shoulders on the floor so that your waist and hips have to do the work!

4 Turn over and decompress your spine as before.

Flexibility Exercises with a Stretch Band

Most people I have given a stretch band to end up almost addicted to it! What I love about the bands is that absolutely anybody can do some sort of exercise with them and you can certainly master exercises which would be inconceivable without them. For example, working the lower abs. A movement you will see in a minute, with legs outstretched and arms over your head, would be almost impossible without a band for anyone but the super-fit. It could hurt your back. But with a stretch band you are supported while being stretched and you can adapt the move as you get stronger; your abs really are taking most of the strain. Then you get results! For now, I just want you to get to appreciate the band as much as I do.

For now, let's see how you hold it.

Any exercise with the stretch band is made slightly harder by shortening your band, increasing resistance. You can either wind it round your hands a couple more times or bring your hands closer together.

Start by holding the band normally, an end in each hand wound once round your hand.

You can also double up the band, which gives the most resistance.

Now stand up straight, or you can sit on a stool without arms or on the floor.

Fold the band in half.

Raise your arms above your head, pulling gently outwards on the band as you do so.

Allow your arms to go backwards as far as you can and if you are able, drop your arms behind your back. Stand or sit up straight and feel the stretch in your shoulders. This is lifting your ribcage, stomach muscles and waist.

Come back to the center and lean slightly to one side. Keep stretching your arms apart. If you are sitting, keep both buttocks on the floor or stool. Hold and breathe. Breathe in and then out as you take your arms up and over to the other side. Breathe evenly.

You can also sit on the center of the band, using its full length. Pick up the left hand side with your right hand and bring the band up the side of your body. You should feel a great stretch in the right side of your waist as the band tries to pull you over to your left. Hold, and then repeat on the other side.

Exercise 1

Lie with your back flat on the floor with your knees in to your chest and the band under the soles of your feet. You might want to wear soft rubber-soled shoes for this – I use bare feet or soft jazz shoes, but you will get less flexibility if you wear sneakers. The stretch band should not slip, and even if it does it won't hurt you.

1 Hold arms in a bicep-curl position.
2 Now stretch out your legs at an angle keeping arms still. Keep your back pressed down to the floor. Bring knees in again and repeat six times. Relax for twenty seconds.
3 Repeat six times.

Exercise 2

1 From the same starting position, this time raise your arms above your head. Do six. Relax for twenty seconds.
2 Repeat six times.

Repeat exercises 1 and 2 again.

Exercise 3

1 From the same starting position, raise your arms high and lift your shoulders off the floor. Hold. Release and repeat six times. Relax for twenty seconds.
2 Repeat.

Exercise 4

1 Place the band under your right foot and hold the ends in your right hand. Stretch the leg up to the ceiling to start, and get a nice hamstring stretch while you are there!
2 Slowly lengthen your leg and reach arm overhead. This stretches your entire side torso and gives you an extra good stretch for your lower abdominal and hip flexor areas.

Do six times, change legs and repeat. Hold each stretch for twenty seconds, trying to extend the stretch all the time.

Exercise 5

1 Turn over onto your front. Double the band and hold as pictured below. Breathe in.
2 Breathe out as you lift your head and shoulders from the floor, extending and pulling the band wide as you do so. You won't go far.
3 Hold for a few seconds, then relax back to the floor. Try to lift and hold even further each time.

This exercise is wonderful for posture and will strengthen and tone your back muscles.

Frequency of Exercise

Never work the same muscles two days running.
What I suggest you do, not just for your first five days but
for the future, is a weekly program along these lines:

Day 1 Full program of toning and stretch band exercises,
plus 45-minute run or walk.

Day 2 30-minute swim, Pilates, or whole body workout.

Day 3 50-minute workout. Attend an aerobics class or use
an aerobics video.

Day 4 Full program of abdominal and stretch band exercises.

Day 5 45-minute run or walk.

Days 6 and 7 Rest, but keep moving. Gentle walking,
sports or household jobs.

Your Posture Is Terrible!

There is no point in losing weight if you are going to ruin the effect by slouching. Exercising your body to perfection, dieting yourself into the ground, and spending a fortune on clothes are a waste of time and money if your chest droops, your neck caves in and your stomach sticks out – all because you don't stand properly.

Good posture is most noticeable when you don't have it. Not only is it important for your look—bad posture suggests depression, lack of confidence, boredom – but it affects your digestion, breathing and general health. Bad posture places strain on ligaments and muscles leading to pain, stiffness, and general lack of mobility.

Nearly everything we do pulls our bodies inward and downward, contributing to poor posture. We are designed to face one way and all our movements lead in that direction – inward and downward. We bend down, lean forward. We have no occasion to lean backward, or to carry out a task with our hands behind our backs. We were meant to live on all fours.

I was standing at the supermarket checkout the other day behind a woman who had a trim bottom encased in skintight jeans, a snug T-shirt and who held great promise of being just as gorgeous from the front. When she finally turned round, my jaw nearly dropped open because she had a particularly prominent stomach. This was not just your average little bulge, and she clearly was not pregnant. Her chest slouched down to her navel, her bust hung unattractively and her stomach protruded. And this was all down to posture.

Good posture is a habit. One of the worst things you can do is to stand for a long time. The natural tendency when standing is to lean backwards, but this conjures up pictures of slanting bodies that look as if they are compensating for a stiff breeze. What we do is stick our hips forward and balance the top half of our body on top of our pelvis, so the socket joints of our hips are taking all the strain of the pelvis. Do it and you will see what I mean. This pushes your stomach forward and there you have your sticking-out stomach. It takes a conscious effort to pull yourself back into alignment, but conscious effort is what the 5-Day program is all about. On the following page you can see the typical backward lean of the body at rest. It causes what is known as "kyphosis."

Kyphosis

Rounded shoulders are often the result of tight chest muscles, which can be the result of slumping over a desk all day or of overdeveloping them with a gym routine. Many women work their pectoral muscles into the ground in the expectation of getting perkier boobs, but this pulls the shoulders forward and can cause a hunched back. Look at bodybuilders' shoulders and back, which tend to be extremely rounded.

Note the effect on the abdomen.

The Dowager's Hump

Despite the name, this problem is increasingly being seen in young people. I recently met a 24-year-old with dowager's hump. She was slim, but you would not have guessed. There was nothing physically wrong with her, either. Over the years she had neglected her physical fitness to such an extent that her back and abdominal muscles had no tone whatever. Her entire weight was sitting on her pelvis. Her back bowed and her stomach looked huge. This postural fault starts with a jutting chin and the upper spine curves to compensate.

Apart from your hairstyle and weight, nothing is more ageing than poor posture. Rightly or wrongly, we associate stooped figures with old people, and next time you see someone who seems young for their age, make a note of what it is about them that gives this impression. It is not just good skin, hair or slimness. A sprightly step and a good carriage are what mark people out as looking younger. A sagging stomach suggests neglect, fatigue and a generally lackluster attitude to life. We have all seen women in their twenties looking like this. Standing properly lifts your ribcage and flattens your stomach.

The Lifetime Maintenance Program

After your 5-Day plan, you are probably feeling great and you want to keep that feeling going. With the Maintenance Program, you can. But it's time for a bit of reality. If this has been a simple program to help you lose those vanity pounds (the ones only you know are there!) that's fine. If you just wanted to banish bloating, I hope you have learned a few tricks. If ever you feel bloated, think about what you have been eating and try to identify your particular culprits and avoid including these in your own cooking. If, however, you need to lose weight and this is a big undertaking, you need to look at a few other aspects of your life.

And the great news is that you don't have to eat yogurt forever or save fruit until the evening. If you have a special date, fine: you know what to do. My Maintenance Program, on the other hand, allows a sensible, controlled diet so you can still lose weight at the same time as keeping your bottom line in view on a daily basis. A too-strict diet would be hard to manage, but the Maintenance Program allows a little leeway within your five steps.

The 5-point Lifetime Maintenance Plan

Having been on the receiving end of thousands of letters and emails from my readers over the years, and having been a private diet counselor to many women, I have often heard the phrase "Where am I going wrong?" It usually comes after yet another diet has failed, although as I said at the beginning of this book, diets can't fail. It is like saying a car is fast—it all depends on who drives it.

Where people go wrong is in not having a proper plan. A diet sheet with a list of meals isn't going to get you through the next crisis or relationship break-up. A few breakfast ideas won't motivate you back onto your diet after a binge. Your problem is still there. So I have devised a 5-point plan that goes beyond the diet to provide a lifetime program to deal with your weight problems.

1 Start again – get rid of the past.
2 Define your bottom line – who do you want to be?
3 Set your midline – what you are going to do to achieve it?
4 Tell somebody that you want to change. Ask for their support.
5 Congratulate yourself – every day.
   Give thanks that you have learned to respect your body,
   what you eat and how you treat yourself.

1 Starting Again

I already talked about getting rid of the past: It's like moving into a new house. You want to chuck out all the old junk and get your new stuff in. You have to do this in your head, too.

Forget wallowing in childhood problems, dreadful parents or school bullying. They were awful but you can't do anything about them now. Don't let them mess up the future. The past was once the future and you did not know what was coming. The future will soon be the past, so don't make it something you look back on and wish it could have been different. Change your past now by changing your future.

Say your farewells to the old you. It sounds cheesy, but some people find it helps to write a letter to themselves saying goodbye. Imagine you are saying this to a friend who is going away. Or maybe you ar ending a relationship and this is your letter to your soon-to-be ex. Go on, write yourself a letter. You can even post it! It will be in complete confidence and you can be anonymous, but at least you will have told somebody.

If this sounds like the worst kind of psycho-babble, believe me – I am the last person to indulge in that sort of thing. I am a practical, down-to-earth sort of woman. But having seen the effect this "farewell" can have on clients of mine, I am happy to recommend it. Who cares what it is called as long as it works for you?

2 So What Is Your Life Really About

So what is your life really about? What do you want, what do you want to achieve or be like? What is your bottom line?

It could be something simple, like "I want to be a size six" or "I want to be healthier." It could be more defined, like "I want a 26-inch waist" or "I don't want to be the fat mother of the bride."

Defining your bottom line is a key stage in your program. It is the reason you are doing it – to change your ways and become a person you are happier with. When things go haywire in the future, let a friend in on the secret and have them ask you, "What's your bottom line?" Repeating it to yourself when you feel low will actually help you get back on track. Write it here:

I . . .

It might seem silly to write here in the book like a schoolgirl, but nobody will see it. And I cannot tell you how useful it will become in the future! Psychologists say that people who stop short of their full weight loss do so because they forget how they felt at the start. It is easy to feel satisfied with less, because the frustration, the anger, the disappointment in yourself, have faded. At any time, you can look back at this page, and seeing your writing will remind you how you felt when you wrote it. It is just a gentle reminder of your ambition for yourself.

3 Set Your Midline

a) What do you have to do?

Losing excess fat is the best thing you can do for your body. Getting a body you love is the pathway to success. Having a permanent, lifestyle diet is common sense. After all, you get a hairstyle which suits you best, a fashion sense and, with any luck, a partner who seems to be a good bet. Why not settle for a personal diet style that keeps you slim without your having to think about it?

A midline is what you have to do – the bare minimum that you are prepared to stick to for the rest of your life – new habits if you will. Basically, there is a set of rules that you are already familiar with which are the basis for success. These include:

- eat regularly
- eat slowly
- chew all food to a paste before swallowing
- eat smaller meals
- eat only at a table
- have fruit as an evening snack
- drink a glass of water after every visit to the restroom
- don't eat when stressed or argumentative
- practice good posture daily
- exercise in some way for at least 45 minutes, five days a week
- do abdominal exercises three times a week.

b) Dropping below the line

Dropping below your midline can also be described as "cheating" or "falling off the wagon" or maybe just "forgetting yourself." It might not be major. But if you are intending to devote your life to looking good you have to know and admit when you have let yourself down. I do not want to sound fixated and obsessed at this point, but if you applied this principle to your work it would make

sense. Skimping on a report, sneaking home early, sliding in late – it's all a bit below-the-midline of what is expected of you. It happens all the time with my clients and it usually results in overeating and weight gain. Try these reasons for dropping below the line:

- I was away from home on a business trip – nothing was normal.
- I was stressed.
- Someone died.
- My pet was ill.
- My children were acting up.
- It was my hormones.
- I'm going through menopause and it's hell.
- I'm unhappy at work.
- My relationship is a mess.

Now this is difficult. All those circumstances are triggers. They are genuine triggers. But if you wait for everything to go right you might as well wait forever, because it isn't going to happen. You and I know that hardly a week goes by when everything is perfect. So you need to get systems in place for eating and managing your diet so your relationship with food carries on as usual when everything around you is chaos. But you can still build in some flexibility. Your limitations can be something like this:

- On business trips, I will have whatever is available on the menu, but no desserts. Although chips and bread are below the line, it's OK if I have one or the other, but not both.
- When my hormones kick in and I give in to cravings, I will just have raw vegetables—they are not supposed to be on my program, but they are better than ice cream or chips!

- When I am a guest I will eat what I am given and if it is 2% milk or sugary cereal, I won't make a fuss, go hungry or eat less when I get home.
- I can have three drinks a day on special occasions, but no more.

Add your own below-the-line get-out clauses, but recognize that they are the exception, not the rule!

c) Going above the line

Going one better than your rules is a short step to diet mania. It is easily done. You eat less one day, your weight dips and you are thrilled. You think that by eating even less you can speed that weight loss on its way. Don't!

This is not above the line or even good. If you have an encouraging weight loss one week, you will have another one the next week. Do not reward yourself by withholding food; do a bit extra for yourself instead, like:

- try out a new healthy gourmet recipe
- buy something new to wear
- dress stylishly to enhance your new figure
- practice walking and sitting elegantly to show off your body and clothes
- buy better food instead of microwave meals.

Write down a few ideas. For example, you might once have thought shellfish and melon was a silly little meal that could not fill anyone up, but now you want something a little better than a potato. Readers often tell me that they had never craved avocado or could not imagine yogurt as a satisfying snack, but now they are hooked. Be prepared to amaze yourself and cook up something special.

d) Falling out of line

I hope you don't find yourself in this place. Overeating happens to all of us, but distinguishing between what is acceptable and what is not is a vital lesson.

Food is precious. Whatever your shortcomings, unhappiness or stresses, many people have nothing to eat and we are lucky to have plenty. Overeating by finishing off a pint of ice cream or having a couple of cookies is one thing; bingeing is another. Bingeing is never acceptable and you should not hand over responsibility for this bad habit by blaming circumstances. *You know what is right and what is wrong.*

Overeating immobilizes you. You become locked in your own world where you think about nothing but food and nobody but yourself. Eating to escape loneliness, anxiety, sadness or dissatisfaction with your life are characterized by:

- letting your self-image slip
- telling lies about what you have eaten
- looking for escapes
- blowing up at people
- making excuses for yourself
- blaming others for your lapses.

What you must do

1 Phone someone and talk about something else. Remove yourself from the situation.
2 Look at your bottom line statement and remind yourself how you felt when you wrote it.
3 Forget what you ate. Wallowing in self-pity is wrong.
4 Match every excuse to a solution – it's OK to have reasons for bad things, but make sure you have a positive solution to end on. For example, "I got stuck in traffic and was too late to exercise" translates to, "I'll leave earlier tomorrow."
5 Get back on your midline tomorrow and do not look back.

Everyone falls out of line sometimes. However, it is not a good place to be and you do not want to go there if you can avoid it. *You can avoid it.*

4 Tell Somebody

Tell somebody that you have decided to change. It is no different from deciding to give up being a businesswoman for another career.

You have every right to a makeover, so tell somebody that you are taking yourself in hand and would appreciate his or her support. Make them realize that this is serious. You have not been happy for some time with the way you eat, your lack of discipline, your health and fitness. Tell somebody that you are trying a new way but you don't want to make a big thing about it. If they are a good friend, they will understand.

The final part of this step is, *Don't go on about it.* This is not a slimming club where you band together and chat about how much chocolate you managed not to eat. Keep it to yourself and get on with it.

5 Congratulate Yourself

The 5-Day program is not easy. You will often see friends out having a good time, knocking back drinks and enjoying a takeout. You can't do this. So how do you cope when things seem unfair and how can you congratulate yourself for your self-denial?

Well, for a start, you certainly aren't denying yourself anything except bad health, bad breath and a hangover. Anyway, you have been denying yourself a lot of good things for a long time: nice clothes, smaller sizes, compliments, confidence, self-esteem . . . it's a long list. Denying yourself a cake or some chocolate or a few vodka tonics, on the other hand, is a feeling that lasts a few minutes. Congratulate yourself that you have seen the difference!

Then there is the tricky question of those lucky friends who can eat and drink to their heart's content and get away with it. They break all the diet rules, live on junk and look like a million dollars. Well, I have met these people too and they rarely look good for long. Anyway, we all have different talents and this is how you must see it. Some people sail through exams while others struggle. Some girls have fantastic hair without trying while others need every conditioner on the market. You can grow your nails long and some people never manage. So what?

Stop thinking about what other people do – this is about YOU.

Think about who you are. You want a flat stomach, you want a slim body and you want to lose weight or keep the figure you have. These are all admirable ambitions because they mean you are taking care of yourself and have pride in your appearance. Losing excess weight is the best thing you can do for your body. Feeling slim and confident will open doors. Congratulate yourself that you are willing to work at it.

Keep Up the Good Work

You have only done five days of this diet so far, but you will have already found that not only does it work, that your stomach is feeling much, much flatter, but that you need less food on your plate. If you want to continue the diet for a further five days, go back to Day 1 and repeat the diet faithfully, or substitute a new evening meal or lunch each day from the recipe section. *All* the meals in this book are suitable for your diet; it is the size of *portion* that matters most in weight loss.

Try also to make or buy the best food you can afford. It need not cost a lot. Do insist on only eating pure, "honest" food without a lot of chemicals added. Get a few great habits, like making your own bread. I make all my own simply because I will not allow manufacturers to push all those chemicals and bloating additives down my throat. It is *not* a chore because I make a huge quantity and freeze it, so I only bake once every few months. My unbleached white bread is famous among my friends, and I have given you a good recipe for it.

Keep Exercising!

Your figure is important to you. That flat stomach feels wonderful. If you give up now, you'll be holding in your stomach for the rest of your life, choosing seats where your stomach is best hidden, wearing clothes you hate. You don't want to feel like that. For the sake of a little self-discipline you can have the body of your dreams, *every* day!

No diet can exercise your muscles. Fat loss won't mobilize your joints. See exercise for its own sake, not as some calorie-burning procedure. The calories you eat are for your health and growth and the calories you burn are for your cardio health.

If it is dark and cold and raining outside you might be tempted to stay in by the fire. *Don't!* The fire is all the better to come back to if you have been out at a fitness class or playing a game of tennis or even walking to the mailbox. Losing weight is fine, but your figure matters too! You don't want to get to summer and find that you're ashamed of your stomach because it's still flabby, despite having lost all that weight.

Eating Out

When You Are a Guest

1 Never say you're on a diet, as it just invites people to make a comment.

2 Never say "only a little, please" or "just a small portion for me," as it alerts people to the fact that you're being careful. Take whatever you are given, eat your usual smaller portion and enjoy it.

3 Never worry about leaving food. You don't owe anybody an explanation of why you are not eating something, and if you are asked if the meal was all right, smile very brightly and say "Yes thank you, it was delicious!"

4 Try not to have second helpings, except if etiquette demands that you keep another diner company.

5 Don't refuse anything unless you genuinely don't like it. Once everyone is into the swing of the evening they won't have a clue whether you've eaten it or not.

When You Are the Hostess

1 People will expect you to be busy, so I doubt that they will notice if you are eating less in comparison or wonder about it if they do. Don't comment on anybody else's eating habits – they could have a problem they'd rather not broadcast and could be embarrassed by close questioning, however well meant.

2 Never eat something simply because it's there. You aren't starving, and mustn't act as if you'll never get the chance to eat a certain dish ever again. Tell yourself that you can have it any time you want it, but not today. Tell yourself that if you still want it tomorrow, you'll have some then.

THE
Maintenance
Diet

I call this my "Free Range" diet because you have more choices. However, don't let this be an excuse to be let off the leash and undo all your good work. This program works, but you can't cheat your body and decide to have takeout one night or overdo the spices. Takeout and flat stomachs just don't mix.

However, I know how great it feels to look forward to a tasty dinner, so I've upped the interest for your Maintenance regime. There are some great ideas on the daily menus but pick and choose from the recipes (p 89) to suit yourself. But remember, if a flat stomach is crucial tonight, go back to the 5 day plan today.

Otherwise you are permitted:
■ two glasses of wine or champagne every day, or one glass of beer or lager
■ bread—as long as it is not wholemeal and is unbleached flour
■ fruit during the day if you wish

Remember:
■ watch the salt
■ practice portion control. Portion size is crucial to any weight loss program. Use the guidelines on page 40.

Please do not forget that your water intake today and every day should be 8 glasses (2 liters). Drink water during the day at every opportunity. Keep a water bottle at your desk or in your bag.

day 1

* Asterisk indicates recipe included in back of book

Breakfast
Oatmeal ($^1/_4$ cup oats and water) served with nonfat milk and honey, if desired
OR
Rice Krispies ($^1/_2$ cup) with nonfat milk

Mid-morning
Small cup coffee with nonfat milk, no sugar
OR
Banana smoothie ($1^1/_4$ cup nonfat milk blended with a banana)

Lunch
Home-made soup (spinach, asparagus or watercress)
WITH
Small protein rich mixed green salad (throw in strips of lean ham or tuna)
OR
Diced half avocado and 4 shrimps, bound with either sour cream and chives
OR
2 tbsp hummus
WITH
1 slice unbleached white bread

Mid-afternoon
Small serving (6 oz) yogurt
OR
Glass (10 oz) nonfat milk

Dinner
Poached, grilled, pan-fried or oven-roasted salmon fillet
WITH
Fava beans and parmesan (4 tbsp)*
Small baked potato (4 oz)
OR
Spaghetti Bolognese* with colorful mixed green salad

Dessert
Poached pear drizzled with chocolate sauce

Late Evening (if hungry)
1 apple or banana, 6 almonds or Brazil nuts, glass warm nonfat milk with 1 tsp honey

day 2

Breakfast

Oatmeal ($\frac{1}{4}$ cup oats and water) served with nonfat milk and honey, if desired

OR

French Toast (2 slices unbleached toast, soaked in 2 beaten eggs, sprayed with oil and fast-grilled or pan-fried)

Mid-morning

Small cup coffee with nonfat milk, no sugar

OR

Banana smoothie ($1\frac{1}{4}$ cup nonfat milk blended with a banana)

Lunch

Cottage cheese and fruit platter (slices of mango, papaya and pineapple)

OR

Cold salmon fillet with dill cream

WITH

Mixed bell pepper, carrot and toasted pine nut salad

Mid-afternoon

Small serving (6 oz) yogurt

OR

Glass (10oz) nonfat milk

Dinner

Plain smoked salmon and cream cheese fluffy omelette
(made with 2 egg yolks and 4 egg whites)

WITH

Side of peas, fava beans and salt-free sweetcorn

OR

Chicken breast with tarragon and parsley
Served on a bed of 2 tbsp organic brown rice

WITH

Spinach and broccoli

Dessert

Grapes with sour cream and brown sugar*

Late Evening (if hungry)

1 apple, 6 almonds or Brazil nuts, glass warm nonfat milk, with 1 tsp honey

day 3

Breakfast
1 egg, scrambled, served on 1 slice unbleached white toast
OR
Rice Krispies (1/2 cup) with nonfat milk

Mid-morning
Small serving (2/3 cup) cottage cheese with celery sticks
OR
Small serving (6 oz) yogurt

Lunch
Spanish omelette*
OR
Cold chicken and avocado salad

Mid-afternoon
Bowl of sliced banana and apple
OR
Glass (10 oz) nonfat milk

Dinner
Salmon with almond and honey crust* with mashed potatoes
(6 oz mashed with non-fat milk, no butter), and
2–3 green vegetables, steamed
OR
Nuts and Bolts Pasta Salad*

Dessert
Rice pudding*

Late Evening (if hungry)
1 apple or 1 banana, 6 almonds or Brazil nuts, glass warm nonfat milk with 1 tsp honey

day 4

Breakfast
Rice Krispies (1/2 cup) with nonfat milk
OR
Boiled egg, 1 slice buttered toast

Mid-morning
Small serving (6 oz) yogurt
OR
Melba toast with cream cheese

Lunch
Caesar salad with small roll and butter
OR
Avocado and pine nut salad

Mid-afternoon
Glass (10 oz) nonfat milk
OR
Banana Smoothie (1 1/4 nonfat milk blended with a banana)

Dinner
Thai Noodle Medley*
OR
Spaghetti alla Carbonara*
WITH
Side dish of mixed, steamed French beans and broccoli

Dessert
Fruit salad (strawberries, blueberries, and sliced grapes),
served with 1 tbsp sour cream or fromage frais

Late Evening (if hungry)
1 apple or 1 banana, 6 almonds or Brazil nuts
Glass warm nonfat milk with 1 tsp honey

day 5

Breakfast
Rice Krispies (1/2 cup) with nonfat milk
OR
Oatmeal (1/4 cup oats and water) served with nonfat milk and honey, if desired

Mid-morning
Melba toast with cream cheese
OR
Small serving (2/3 cup) cottage cheese with celery sticks

Lunch
Homemade soup (spinach, asparagus, watercress)
with 1 slice unbleached white bread
OR
Cold diced chicken breast with diced mango, sour cream, and 2 tbsp steamed rice.
Served on bed of lettuce.
OR
2-3 slices smoked salmon, with 1 tsp sour cream, capers, and lemon
with 1 slice unbleached white bread

Mid-afternoon
1 banana
OR
Glass (10oz) nonfat milk

Dinner
Grilled salmon with tarragon butter*
Served on a bed of spinach
OR
Lemon Paprika Chicken with Walnuts and Bowtie Pasta*

Dessert
Rice pudding

Late Evening (if hungry)
1 apple or 1 banana, 6 almonds or Brazil nuts
Glass warm nonfat milk with 1 tsp honey

24-Hour Emergency Plan

What if you've got just a day or so to look your very best? What if you've suddenly been invited somewhere and want to wear your slinkiest outfit or most figure-hugging dress? Do you spend all day nibbling at bits of fruit?

This isn't a weight-loss diet, but when a flatter stomach is particularly important to you it's easy to fall into the trap of eating nothing all day, or snacking on raw vegetables. This isn't the right approach. So what do you do?

1 Start the day before if you can, and for dinner have a stir-fry with plenty of corn, peas and other fresh vegetables. Drink two or three glasses of water during the evening and have 1½oz (40g) of All-Bran or bran flakes in the late evening, with a few grapes, sliced apple and an orange if possible.

2 On the day itself, drink plenty of water. For breakfast have oatmeal made with 1oz (30g) oats and water served with 1 tsp honey, if desired, and nonfat milk.

3 Throughout the morning, have a tablespoon of yogurt with live and active cultures every hour.

4 For lunch, have a small mixed-green salad with chicken or with half an avocado.

5 Two hours later, drink a glass of nonfat milk.

6 In the late afternoon, have a small mixed-green salad with 1oz (30g) grated cheese or 2 tablespoons of tuna.

Do not eat after this.

This regime works extremely well for just one day, after which you must go back to normal eating.

Recipes

No-Bloat Meals

The 5-Day program is about simplicity. Simple meals are not boring meals. By using the freshest and best ingredients you can afford and obtain, you will care for your body holistically. As a result you will find yourself feeling energetic and positive, functioning better, with better skin, a fat-free body and of course that wonderful non-bloated flat stomach.

This section contains standard no-bloat meals. Use them any time you like on the program. The second section has slightly more ambitious meals which might include a few controversial foods. You might like to save these for non-program days or you might find your body tolerates the ingredients well.

Whatever you decide to do, you can always add items as it suits you, as long as you remember your basic program—sitting down to eat, chewing thoroughly and portion control.

Cooking Methods

Always poach, grill, stir-fry with minimum oil or roast with a tsp. of butter. Never deep-fry or boil out of existence!

Basic Fish Meals

Cod, Halibut, Haddock, Etc.

On the 5-Day program, white fish should be poached in milk or water and served plain on a bed of:
- spinach
- mashed carrots
- mashed parsnips.

White fish can also be baked in the oven in a sauce of canned, chopped tomatoes.

One-step Mediterranean Cod

You can use any white fish for this, especially sea bass or cod. It is simple but incredibly tasty and ideal for the busy person – it will cook while you are taking a shower!

1 fillet fish per person
1 can (14^1/$_2$oz) chopped tomatoes with
    herbs and garlic
1 tsp capers
1 large chopped bell pepper
chopped cilantro or parsley, to serve

Preheat oven to 200°F

Place the fish fillets in an oven-to-table dish. Mix tomatoes, pepper, and capers, and pour over fillets.

Bake in the oven for 20 minutes, until the fish is cooked through.

Serve on a bed of mashed potatoes, rice, or if watching calories, a bed of spinach. Give a few good turns of the sea salt grinder, to taste.

Salade Niçoise

This is a standard tuna fish salad, with hard-boiled egg, cold French beans and a sprinkling of olives.

Layer the salad starting with mixed greens and watercress. Add the other ingredients, finishing with 3^1/$_2$oz (100g) tuna fish.

Feel free to add ingredients as they suit you. Lemon juice or Vinaigrette (page 101) are suitable dressings.

Fish

Salmon with Almond and Honey Crust

Making this dish is like battering a piece of fish!
Serves 2

2 salmon fillets
2 tsp butter
2 tsp honey
1 tbsp skinless flaked almonds, crushed roughly

Preheat the oven to 400°F.

Put the butter and honey in a pot and heat through or place in a dish and microwave until melted and runny.

Place the crushed almonds on a flat plate.

Pat the salmon dry. Dip it into, or brush with, the butter and honey mixture, top side only.

Now firmly press the buttered side of the fish onto the crushed almonds. Pour over any remaining butter mixture.

Place in a greased, ovenproof dish or a throwaway foil tray. Cover with foil and bake for 15 minutes. Then remove the foil to allow the top crust of the fish to crisp (5 minutes).

Crab and Rice Ball Salad

Fragrant Thai rice or sticky paella rice is best for this dish as it sticks easily to form firm balls. You can use either fresh crabmeat or canned.
Serves 3

3 cups cooked rice
1 tbsp vinegar
1 tsp sugar
1 large can crabmeat
1 clove garlic, chopped
1 tbsp chopped lemon grass
1 tbsp fresh grated ginger
2 red Thai chillies seeded and chopped finely
OR 1 tsp dried hot chillies
2 green onions, finely chopped
vegetable oil, for frying

Combine the rice, vinegar and sugar in a bowl.

Drain the crabmeat.

Stir the crab and all the other ingredients, plus the rice. Form into balls, the size of golf balls.

Deep-fry, in batches, in hot oil until browned and crisp. Drain on kitchen paper.

Serve on a bed of mixed romaine lettuce, chicory, rocket.

A tasty dressing for this is horseradish cream. I use my own home-grown horseradish—otherwise buy horseradish cream and mix with a little olive oil, lemon juice and chopped fresh dill or plain sour cream.

Scallop and Bacon Provencale

Serves 2

$^1/_2$ medium onion, finely chopped or grated
1 clove garlic, crushed (optional)
1 cup fresh scallops
1 cup diced smoked bacon
1 chopped red chili
14oz (large can) chopped tomatoes with herbs
salt and fresh-ground black pepper (to taste)
5oz glass dry white wine
4 tbsp steamed rice
small bunch cilantro, roughly torn into shreds
(garnish)

Method
Heat oil in a large pan. Add the onion and garlic and sauté until soft. Remove from pan and set aside.

Add the scallops and bacon and cook over a medium heat, turning occasionally, until cooked through. Remove and set aside.

Return the onions and garlic to the pan and add the wine, chili, tomatoes and seasoning. Simmer for five minutes.

Add back the scallops and bacon and heat through.

Serve garnished with cilantro on a bed of steamed rice. Add a dressed green salad.

Scandinavian Smoked Salmon Potato Cakes with Dill Cream

2 large potatoes
$^1/_2$ lb smoked salmon offcuts or chopped slices
1 tbsp butter
zest and juice of 2 lemons, kept separate
fresh-ground black pepper

For the dill cream
1 tbsp sour cream
1 tbsp snipped fresh dill or tsp dried dill
some of the lemon juice, above

Preheat oven to 400°F

Peel and boil potatoes, mash with a little butter, but do not allow to become soft.

Chop and add the smoked salmon, black pepper, half the lemon zest and cilantro leaves.

Using floured hands, form into small balls, the size of a golf ball. Flatten slightly.

Place the fishcakes on a greased baking sheet; dot the remaining butter into each fishcake.

Place in hot oven for 20-30 minutes, turning once.

To make the dill cream:
Mix the sour cream, lemon zest and snipped dill. Serve 2-3 cakes each on a crisp green salad with a spoon of dill cream.

Beef

On the 5-Day program you are always permitted a small fillet or sirloin steak with salad or spinach. For your evening meals, you may also have other mixed vegetables, especially carrots, parsnips, zucchini, snow peas, snap peas, and string beans.

Chicken

Grilled Chicken in Orange Marinade

Serves 1

1 skinless, boneless chicken breast (4-5oz)
juice and zest of 1 large orange
1 tbsp walnut oil or olive oil
1 clove garlic, crushed (optional)

Place all the ingredients in an ovenproof dish, stir well to mix, cover with foil and refrigerate for at least two hours or overnight, if possible.

Preheat the oven to 350°F. Remove the chicken from the dish and place on a wire rack over a roasting tin in the oven. Cook for about 20 minutes.

Turn the heat to high, and grill the chicken thoroughly on both sides until brown and slightly caramelized.

Alternatively pan-fry with the lid on tightly, over medium heat, turning frequently to prevent burning. This takes about 10 minutes total (5 minutes each side), depending on the thickness of the chicken. Always check that it is thoroughly cooked.

Chicken with Almonds

Serves 4

4 skinless, boneless chicken breasts
packet of sliced almonds (or pine nuts)
oil

Flatten 4 boneless chicken breasts with a rolling pin, after covering the chicken with a piece of wax paper. This avoids tearing the meat.

Scatter a packet of sliced almonds over a dinner plate. Brush the chicken breasts with oil and place on the sliced almonds. Press thoroughly to coat each side.

Fry gently in a pan containing 1 tbsp olive oil, turning once.

Alternatively you can preheat the oven to 400°F and cook on a rack for 20 minutes.

Skinny Chicken and Garden Grill

Serves 4

A perfect local dish or perfectly grilled chicken on a simple salad of pan-fried eggplant, zucchini, tomato, red bell peppers and asparagus topped with parmesan shavings.

4 skinless, boneless chicken breasts
  (6oz), flattened
2 zucchini, sliced into julienne strips
1 eggplant, sliced into rounds
12 asparagus spears
2 bell peppers de-seeded and sliced
1 tbsp olive oil
Few parmesan shavings (optional)
2 tsp toasted sesame seeds (optional),
  to decorate
1 tsp soy sauce

Heat the olive oil in the pan until hot but not smoking. Add the chicken, put lid on and turn heat to medium. Cook for five minutes each side and test that it is cooked by cutting into the breast. It should be white throughout without a hint of pink.

Remove chicken from pan and set aside. Add another tsp of olive oil to the pan, turn heat up and add the vegetables. Turn quickly, and keep shaking the pan. Stir-fry swiftly, not allowing the vegetables to stick.

Add 1 tsp soy sauce and shake thoroughly to disperse.

Meanwhile cut the chicken into strips. Turn the vegetables out onto a hot serving dish, top with the chicken and the parmesan shavings. Add a few sesame seeds, if you wish, to decorate.

Chicken with Watermelon and Hazelnut Salad (and Raspberry Vinaigrette)

This dish makes plain grilled chicken suddenly sensational. Save time by having raspberry vinaigrette and toasted hazelnuts always in your pantry. You can substitute cranberries for raspberries.
Serves 1

1 skinless, boneless chicken breast per person
1/3 cup toasted hazelnuts
1/2 medium seedless watermelon
mixed greens
1 cup fresh raspberries
1/2 tbsp olive oil

Raspberry vinaigrette
1 cup raspberries
1/2 cup hazelnut oil
1/4 cup raspberry vinegar

First, process all the vinaigrette ingredients until pureed. Pour through a sieve to get rid of the seeds.

To toast hazelnuts, either put them into a hot oven, without any oil, constantly shaking OR put into a dry large frying pan and keep shaking as they gradually turn brown. Take away from heat and leave—(they will keep cooking in their own oil and be extremely hot to touch, so be careful).

Grill the chicken with a drizzle of oil, until cooked through.

Cut the watermelon into chunks. Combine in a bowl with the raspberries and lettuce.

Slice the chicken thinly or dice, drizzle with the vinaigrette and sprinkle with the nuts. Combine gently with all the other ingredients and serve.

Moroccan Chicken Salad

Serves 2

1 tbsp Moroccan spice mix
2 tbsp olive oil
2 skinless, boneless chicken breasts
1 medium eggplant
2 large prepared bell peppers (canned or in jars)
2 cups water
2 cups couscous
1/2 cup shelled pistachios, toasted
1/4 cup fresh cilantro leaves
1/4 cup fresh chopped mint

Moroccan dressing
1/4 cup lemon juice
1 tbsp grated lemon zest
1/2 cup olive oil
2 cloves garlic, crushed
8 cardamom pods, bruised
1 tsp cumin seeds, toasted
pinch ground turmeric

Combine spices, 1 tbsp oil and add the chicken to coat. Leave to marinade for 30 minutes

Chop whole eggplant, quarter peppers.

Cook the chicken in the hot oil until browned all over and cooked through. Set aside.

Using same oil, or add a little more, cook the eggplant until browned.

Put the couscous in a bowl, cover with the 2 cups boiling water and allow to stand. When the water is absorbed, fluff the couscous with a fork.

Gently toss the chicken, eggplant, peppers, couscous, pistachios, mint and cilantro with the dressing.

To make dressing
Simply combine all the ingredients in a screw-top jar and shake well. A serving is two good tablespoons. Add a side green salad.

Lemon Paprika Chicken with Walnuts and Bowtie Pasta

Serves 2

2 skinless, boneless chicken breasts
8oz bowtie pasta (farfalle)
grated rind and juice of a lemon
$1/2$ cup olive oil
1 clove garlic, crushed
1 tsp sweet paprika
1 tsp ground turmeric
$1/2$ cup broken walnuts
1 small cucumber, peeled and sliced into ribbons with a vegetable peeler
vegetable oil, for frying
1 tbsp vinegar
a little sour cream, to combine

Combine chicken breasts, paprika, olive oil, garlic, lemon rind and juice and turmeric in a large bowl. Allow to marinate an hour or if you can, overnight. Turn chicken a couple of times.

Combine the cucumber ribbons with the walnuts and vinegar.

Meanwhile, take out the chicken from the turmeric marinade. Cook in a large heated pan with a little oil, until browned all over and cooked through.

Cook the pasta according to directions. Drain and put immediately into a serving dish and keep warm.

Slice the chicken, add to the pasta with the cucumber and walnuts, add the sour cream and mix. Serve straight away with a side dish of crisp sweetcorn and peas.

Greek Chicken Salad

Serves 4

4 skinless, boneless chicken breasts
1 large romaine lettuce, chopped
1 bunch mint
6oz (170g) blueberries

For the dressing
$1/2$ pint (300ml) Greek yogurt
1 tsp brown sugar
1 tsp ground cumin
juice of 1 lemon
1 tbsp olive oil

Grill or charcoal grill the chicken breasts and arrange down the center of a serving plate.

Combine all the dressing ingredients in a bowl and beat well. Stir in most of the blueberries, reserving a few to scatter garnish.

Surround the chicken with the lettuce and mint sprigs.

Spoon the dressing generously over the chicken and scatter with the blueberries and chopped mint.

Vegetarian

Caesar Salad v

Serves 2

1 tbsp mayonnaise
1 garlic clove, crushed
1 slice thick-cut stale bread
1 tsp vegetable oil
1 romaine lettuce, separated into leaves
1oz (30g) Parmesan cheese, coarsely grated

Mix the garlic into the mayonnaise.

Make the croutons by cutting the bread into half-inch cubes. Heat the oil until very hot and fry the cubes quickly until golden brown, which will take a couple of minutes. Remove with a slotted spoon and blot dry with kitchen paper.

Add the cooled croutons and the mayonnaise to the lettuce and toss together. Sprinkle the Parmesan cheese over the salad and serve.

Wild Rice and Pecan Salad v

Serves 2
One serving is 4 tablespoons

1 cup cooked and drained wild rice
1 tbsp butter
1 clove garlic, crushed (optional)
2 cups mushrooms (white button)
2 tbsp red wine
3 celery sticks
1 cup pecans, halved
$1/2$ cup raisins
Grated rind and juice of an orange
$1/2$ cup olive oil

Heat butter in a large pan, add the garlic and mushrooms and fry gently. Add the red wine and the rice and heat through so the wine is absorbed.

Cut celery into matchsticks, put into a serving bowl with the nuts, raisins and other ingredients. Add the rice mixture and toss gently to combine.

Serve hot or cold in a picnic or as a cold lunchbox.

Cannelloni Stuffed with Spinach and Almonds v

This makes enough for 4-6 servings. I suggest you either have your own small portion, or use this for quick re-heated meals during the week, as it keeps quite well, covered, in the refrigerator for 5-7 days.

Despite the cream content, a small portion of this, served with a crisp salad or fava beans, will make a lowfat, low calorie dinner or light lunch.

12–16 sheets or tubes of cannelloni
2 lbs leaf spinach or large pack frozen spinach
2 tbsp butter
1 cup ground almonds
2 tbsp heavy cream
Sea salt and fresh ground black pepper (to taste)
¹/₂ cup grated unprocessed gruyere cheese
1 cup light cream
¹/₂ cup grated Parmesan cheese

Preheat the oven to 300°F

Cook the cannelloni until a little underdone. If using ready-to-use pasta, ignore this step.

Put 1 tsp butter in a large pan, melt and add the spinach. Cook fast, shaking the pan, until the spinach is half its bulk. This should take less than 3 minutes. If using frozen spinach, ignore this step.

Put the spinach into a bowl; add almonds and remaining butter, heavy cream, seasoning and gruyere cheese. Mix well.

Drain the cannelloni. Lay a portion of the spinach mixture on a sheet and roll. Otherwise stuff the tube with 1 tbsp of the spinach mixture.

Continue filling and rolling, tucking the ends so they are underneath. Grease a large shallow ovenproof dish and lay the cannelloni in side by side, so they fit snugly.

Pour the single cream over, sprinkle with parmesan and bake for 20 minutes. The cannelloni should be heated through and the cheese melted. Sprinkle with toasted flaked almonds and serve piping hot.

Herb, Cheese or Spanish Omelette v

All types of omelettes are good non-bloat dishes. Use three eggs per person and 1 tsp of butter in the pan. For a herb omelette, add a mixture of herbs to taste. For a cheese omelette, add 15g (1/2oz) grated Cheddar cheese.

For a Spanish omelette, add chopped red and green pepper and a few chunks of cold potato.

Spinach omelettes are also good.

Herb Omelette Salad v

Serves 4

4 eggs, beaten
2 tbsp chopped fresh herbs
Salt and freshly ground black pepper
Butter
1 large red pepper, seeded and cut into strips
1 large green pepper, seeded and cut into strips
$^1/_2$ cucumber, cut into thin strips
Vinaigrette (page 101) to taste

Beat the eggs with the herbs and 2 tbsp water. Season with salt and pepper. Heat 1 tsp of butter or margarine in an omelette pan and use the eggs to make two thinly, lightly set omelettes. Turn out on wax paper, roll up and leave to cool slightly.

Toss the remaining ingredients together.

Thinly slice the omelette and scatter over the prepared salad ingredients. Serve immediately.

Baked Cheese Tomatoes v

Serves 1

1oz (30g) grated mature Cheddar cheese
2 large beef tomatoes
1 tbsp breadcrumbs

Preheat the oven to 350°F.

Simply scoop out the middle of the tomatoes and discard the seeds. Fill the cavity with the grated cheese, half in each tomato. Add $^1/_2$ tbsp of breadcrumbs to each tomato.

Using a sharp knife, score through the skin right round the tomato. This will stop the skin splitting.

Bake for 10–15 minutes or grill until the cheese is bubbling and slightly browned.

Sauces and Dressings

Vinaigrette

This keeps for ages in the fridge. The amount you make is up to you, depending on whether you are in a single household or are feeding half a dozen. The proportions are the same:

Use 3 parts olive oil or good vegetable oil to one part wine vinegar.

Pour into a screw-top jar.

Add 2 tsp Dijon mustard, 1 tsp sugar and some coarsely ground black pepper.

If you like garlic, add a crushed clove.

Shake the mixture thoroughly and taste. Adjust to suit your own tastes.

Mayonnaise

Most people who are dieting worry unnecessarily about the high oil content in mayonnaise. The first consideration is that in fresh mayonnaise most of the fat content is good fat—not saturated—and the second is that we use tiny quantities. Use this mayonnaise on your hard-boiled eggs or your cold poached salmon. It will last for up to two days in the fridge. Use either a blender or an electric whisk for this.

1 egg yolk (reserve the white for something else, like cheese soufflé or a meringue)
1 pint (570ml) good oil

Place the egg yolk in a clean bowl and add a few drops of oil, whisking all the time. Continue to add the oil by the drop until it seems that the mixture is amalgamating.

Graduate to pouring the oil in a thin stream, but slowly: If you start to pour the oil too quickly, the mixture will curdle.

Continue pouring, mixing all the time, until the mixture is thick and creamy.

If the mixture curdles, try rescuing it by adding a spoonful of hot water or a small dash of vinegar. If you have spoiled it, however, start again with a fresh yolk and add the curdled mixture, bit by bit.

Now you have a basic mayonnaise. Try a teaspoon of curry powder for curried mayonnaise or the grated zest of a lemon for lemon mayonnaise. Or add some crushed garlic or finely chopped basil leaves.

Homemade Fiery Sundried Tomato Salsa

This is not complicated at all, though it may sound like it could be. Once you have the ingredients, you simply cook them together then divide into jars. It is fantastic with plain homemade burgers, grilled chicken or fish, and livens up low-calorie foods without additives, artificial flavorings or seasonings. It never fails to impress your friends and family.

Makes 2-3 1lb jars

3 cups dry-packed sundried tomatoes
1 tbsp olive oil
2 medium white onions
2 tsp grated ginger
3 tsp mustard seeds
2 tsp mixed spice
3 medium apples, chopped small
1 cup sultanas
1 large papaya, peeled and chopped coarsely
1 cup brown sugar
1 cup balsamic vinegar
$1/2$ cup cider vinegar
2 cups apple juice
**3 fresh, red Thai chilies seeded and chopped
    finely**
**4 red bell peppers, de-seeded and chopped
    quite small**
2 yellow peppers, as above
1 cup water

(Tied in a small old handkerchief or bit of old cotton cloth)
$1/2$ tsp whole allspice
$1/2$ tsp black peppercorns

Put all the vegetables, with the water to coat bottom of pan, in a large heavy-based pan and set on a medium heat to simmer down slowly.

As the mixture begins to soften, add the cloth bag with the ingredients tied tight to prevent them falling out. Let these infuse in the mixture.

Add the sugar and stir slowly. Allow to dissolve for about 5 minutes.

Simmer for about 1 hour, stirring occasionally until mixture thickens. Add the vinegars toward the end. Discard bag of spices.

Spoon the hot salsa into hot sterilized jars, seal while hot.

Desserts

Grapes with Sour Cream and Brown Sugar

Serves 4

1 large bunch seedless red or green grapes
1 cup sour cream
2 tablespoons light brown sugar

Wash grapes, remove from stems. Chill.

Whisk sour cream in a small bowl. Place grapes in serving dishes. Spoon sour cream over grapes and sprinkle with brown sugar.

Rice Pudding

Serves 3–4

I first became enthusiastic about rice pudding when I was pregnant with my second child and had to endure a long journey from the country to town and a freezing mile walk to the hospital for my check-ups. The whole procedure took half a day, but by starting with oatmeal and taking a cup of rice pudding with me I managed it with gusto—not easy when you're trailing a two-year-old.

Since then I have made rice pudding every week, summer or winter, because it is not only nourishing and healthy but it is equally delicious hot or cold. The calorie content is not at all high for a snack, and with the addition of fruit, you will have no need of another meal. Made with nonfat milk it's full of calcium, protein and starch. Try it!

$1/4$ cup short-grain (pudding) rice
1 cup nonfat milk
$1^1/2$ tbsp sugar

Preheat the oven to 350°F.

Combine all the ingredients in a lightly greased pot and cook for 2 hours, stirring occasionally to separate rice grains.

Either eat straight away, hot, with some cinnamon, or refrigerate until needed. It can then be microwaved if you want it hot.

Maintenance
Program Recipes

Once again, these "recipes" are more like cooking methods. The ingredients are simple but delicious.

Grilled Salmon with Tarragon Butter

Serves 1

1 4–6oz (125–180g) salmon fillet
1 tsp butter
fresh tarragon leaves, chopped,
** or a pinch of dried tarragon**
parsley to garnish

Grill the fish with a dot of the butter.

Soften the rest of the butter, combine with the tarragon and place it on the hot fish.

Garnish with parsley and serve immediately with vegetables.

Shrimp Portofino

Serves 1

6oz (cooked weight) farfalle pasta
4oz peeled, cooked shrimps
1 tsp pine nuts
Large handful spinach
¹/₄ oz butter, mixed with zest of a lemon
1 tbsp oil

Heat a large frying pan. Add the pine nuts and toast, without oil, tossing the pan continuously. This should take about 2-3 minutes, but take care—the nuts can burn suddenly!

Turn the pine nuts onto a dish and set aside.

Put the oil into the pan, heat, add the shrimps and heat through, tossing continuously

Add the cooked pasta, pine nuts and spinach. Keep shaking the pan until mixture is heated through. Finally add the lemon butter, remove from the heat and serve immediately with a green salad.

Beef

On the Maintenance program, you may have a small fillet or sirloin steak with salad and other vegetables, including parsnips, carrots, Rutabega and zucchini, squash, sugar snap peas, French beans, and potatoes.

Beef Skewers (Kebabs) with Spicy Salsa

1 filet mignon per person
1 medium pita bread per person

Marinade
1 small onion, chopped finely
1 clove garlic, crushed
¹/₄ cup natural yogurt
1 tbsp lemon juice
1 tbsp olive oil
¹/₄ cup mint leaves shredded
3 tsp white wine vinegar

Cut filets into 1" cubes, thread onto wooden skewers.

Combine the marinade ingredients, place the skewers in marinade, turn, cover and leave in fridge overnight or for 2 hours.

Cook skewers, in batches, in heated oiled pan (or on the grill) until cooked as desired.

Serve with the fiery salsa (p 102) and a crisp green salad or mixed fresh vegetables.

Beef in Red Wine

Serves 4

This dish is not the traditional, standard French dish, but it is a good alternative. I have removed the onion and mushrooms. It still tastes excellent, mostly thanks to the bacon and brandy. Serve with crisp green vegetables (from the list of those allowed) or with young new potatoes or rice. Great when you are entertaining but want to observe your new rules.

1 tsp vegetable oil

1½ lb best stewing or braising steak, cubed
    (leanest braising beef)

1 glass brandy

½ bottle red wine

½ clove garlic, crushed (optional)

6 slices bacon, smoked

1 tbsp cornflour

2 cans chopped tomatoes with added herbs
    and olives

4 tsp tomato purée

add salt, freshly ground black pepper, fresh herbs
    to taste

fresh parsley (preferably flat-leaf)

2 tbsp low-fat sour cream

Preheat the oven to 325°F.

Heat the oil over a moderate heat in a large pan, and add the cubed beef. Keep turning to seal all sides, until all traces of red have gone.

Add the brandy, turn heat high and allow to "flame". Turn down the heat and add the wine and crushed garlic (if using), plus 2 glasses of water. Stir.

Transfer to a casserole dish, put the lid on tightly and cook in the oven for 1½ hours.

Meanwhile, chop and fry the bacon and set aside. When cool, toss in 1 tbsp cornflour and stir to coat. Save.

When the beef comes out of the oven, add the tinned tomatoes and tomato purée. Mix well. Stir in the bacon. Return to the oven for 1 hour.

Remove from the oven and stir well. Add a little more water if needed, but do not make the casserole too wet.

Add salt, pepper and mixed herbs to taste.

Return to the oven to heat through. Just before serving, stir in 2 tbsp half-fat crème fraîche and top with a good sprinkling of coarsely chopped fresh parsley.

Hamburgers

These burgers are easy to make, and I recommend buying extra-lean ground beef. I also suggest asking a butcher to mince prime fillet or tenderloin steak for you. I tend to make several burgers at once and freeze them. If you have a big family or you want to plan ahead for other meals, you might as well do the same!

2 lbs leanest ground steak
1 onion, finely grated or minced (not dried)
Sea salt and fresh ground black pepper
   (to taste)
2 eggs, beaten
2 slices old white bread or bake a fresh loaf
   (best) and leave it out 2 days
1 tbsp mixed paprika, chilli powder and garlic
   granules (optional)
other spices and herbs to suit yourself
1 tbsp any good oil

Using a blender or food processor, make the bread into fine crumbs. (For future use, make crumbs out of old bread and store in freezer. They keep three months.)

   Put the steak into a large mixing bowl. Add the minced or grated onion, beaten eggs, and breadcrumbs. Then add the spices, herbs and all other ingredients, including the oil. Mix thoroughly with your hands.

   Using a burger mold or simply forming into balls and flattening, make burgers no bigger than 4 inches diameter (they will shrink with cooking).

   Grill or barbecue five minutes each side. Serve with fiery sundried tomato salsa (p102).

Spiced Lamb Salad with Mango Dressing

First get your spices sorted: I recommend making a larger amount and keeping in a screw-top jar, to save labor next time to make this delicious dish!

2 tbsp ground cumin
2 tbsp ground cilantro
1 tbsp ground turmeric
1 tsp hot paprika
2 tsp garlic salt
1 lb loin of lamb or lamb cutlets
1 medium red and one yellow bell pepper,
   sliced thinly
1 onion, sliced thinly
2 medium avocados, sliced thinly
lettuce and cilantro leaves

Mango dressing
1 cup canned mango puree
juice of a lime

Simply mix the ingredients in a screw-top jar, shake and serve.

Place the lamb in a bowl with as much of the spice mix as you would like to use, for personal preference. Keep the rest for another time. Roll until all sides are covered, leave for 30 minutes up to overnight.

   Cook the lamb in shallow oil until browned all over and to the pinkness you prefer. Rest 5 minutes then slice thinly.

   Mix the lamb with the peppers, onion, avocado, lettuce, and cilantro, drizzle with dressing and serve.

Smoked Salmon with Pasta, Watercress and Dill

Serves 1

2oz (60g) dry pasta shapes
1 slice smoked salmon cut into strips
(or about 3^1/$_2$oz/100g ready sliced)
few fronds of snipped fresh dill or a pinch of
dried dill
1 large bunch watercress, stems removed
freshly ground black pepper
1 tsp sour cream

Boil the pasta until cooked. Drain and return to the pan.

Keeping the heat under the pan very low, add the smoked salmon and stir through quickly. The salmon will go pale as it cooks.

Straight away, add the dill and watercress. Mix thoroughly, then add the sour cream and black pepper. Taste for seasoning. (The salmon is very salty, so don't add any salt.)

Serve immediately on very hot plates, as pasta goes cold very quickly.

Spaghetti Bolognese

Serves 2

^{1}/$_2$ lb of extra-lean ground beef
1^1/$_2$ tbsp olive oil
1 small onion, finely chopped
1 clove garlic, crushed (optional)
8oz (225g) canned chopped tomatoes with herbs
1 tbsp concentrated tomato purée
1 lb (8oz) dry spaghetti
few leaves fresh oregano or ^{1}/$_2$ tsp dried
oregano
salt and freshly ground black pepper
Parmesan cheese

In a large frying pan, cook beef without added fat or oil, and until any fat runs clear. Drain. Set the meat aside.

Heat the oil and gently sauté the onion until softened. Drain off any excess oil and add the meat, garlic, tomatoes and tomato paste. Turn down the heat, cover the pan and simmer for 5 minutes.

Cook the spaghetti as directed on the packet.

Add the oregano to the meat mixture. Stir and taste. Season if necessary. Drain the spaghetti and add the mince mixture to the pasta and toss.

Sprinkle with Parmesan cheese and serve with a green salad.

Spaghetti Alla Carbonara

Serves 4

1 lb spaghetti
4 eggs
1 tsp black pepper
3 tsp Pecorino Romano, plus extra, for serving
2 tsp cream (optional)
3 tsp extra-virgin olive oil
3 slices pancetta

Boil the spaghetti in salted water until it is al dente. Drain and set aside.

Beat the eggs. Add the black pepper and cheese to the beaten eggs. Set aside. Add cream to this mixture, if desired, for a creamier dish.

Put the oil in a saucepan with the pancetta, and sauté for 5 minutes. Add the spaghetti into the pan and sauté for another 3 minutes.

Turn off the flame (this is important) and add the egg and cheese mixture to the pasta and mix. Serve with additional Pecorino Romano on top.

Pasta Primavera v

Serves 4

3 carrots, peeled and cut into thin strips
2 medium zucchini, cut into thin strips
2 yellow squash, cut into thin strips
1 onion thinly sliced
1 yellow bell pepper, cut into thin strips
1 red bell pepper, cut into thin strips
¼ cup olive oil
Kosher salt and freshly ground pepper
1 tbsp dried Italian herbs or herbes de
   Provence
1 pound farfalle (bowtie pasta)
15 cherry tomatoes, halved
½ cup grated Parmesan

Preheat oven to 400°F.

On a large heavy baking sheet, toss all of the vegetables with the oil, salt, pepper, and dried herbs to coat. Transfer half of the vegetable mixture to another heavy large baking sheet and arrange evenly over the baking sheets. Bake until the carrots are tender and the vegetables begin to brown, stirring after the first 10 minutes, about 20 minutes total.

Meanwhile, cook the pasta in a large pot of boiling salted water until al dente, tender but still firm to the bite (about 8 minutes). Drain, reserving 1 cup of the cooking liquid.

Toss the pasta with the vegetable mixtures in a large bowl to combine. Toss with the cherry tomatoes and enough reserved cooking liquid to moisten. Season the pasta with salt and pepper, to taste. Sprinkle with the Parmesan and serve immediately.

Thai Noodle Medley

This dish is easier than it sounds! Once you have the sauce made it can stay in the refrigerator up to a week until you need it.

12 oz package rice noodles
$^1/_2$ cup carrots in thin strips
$^1/_2$ cup red bell peppers in strips
$^1/_2$ cup broccoli florets parboiled and chilled

Sauce
1 garlic clove, crushed
a few gratings of fresh ginger, doesn't matter how much
2 chopped scallions
2 tbsp smooth peanut butter
8 oz firm tofu, diced
1 tsp dark sesame oil
$^1/_4$ cup honey
$^1/_4$ cup light soy sauce
$^1/_4$ cup rice wine vinegar
pinch ground red pepper

Mix all the sauce ingredients together by hand, in processor, or just pour into a screw-top jar and shake well.

Prepare noodles according to package instructions. Drain and cool. Pour into a large bowl and put the chilled sauce over. Toss to coat.

Add the raw vegetables, toss again and serve.

Dry-Roast Oven Chips

These could not be more simple or more tasty. You'll wonder why you ever wanted roast potatoes or potato chips!

1 large (8oz) potato
Sea salt

Turn oven high.

Microwave the large potato for three minutes. Allow to cool a little, so the steam does not scald when you cut open the potato.

Cut potato, skin on, into quarters. Then cut each quarter into further halves. This should make thick chip-style pieces. Roll in sea salt, which you have sprinkled on a piece of paper or a plate.

Put into the very hot oven, on a baking tray or foil dish, and cook, turning once or twice, for about 20-30 minutes, until the edges are crisp and the potato soft to the fork.

Serve immediately, as they go soft quickly.

Nuts and Bolts Pasta Salad

Serves 4

2 oz tricolor corkscrew pasta (rotini)
2 oz wheel-shaped pasta (rotelle)
1 cup frozen mixed vegetables
¼ cup plain lowfat yogurt
2 tbsp Parmesan cheese
1 tbsp mayonnaise
1 tbsp milk
½ tsp garlic powder

Cook pasta in boiling water for 10 minutes; add frozen vegetables and cook for 2 minutes more. Drain, rinse, and cool to room temperature.

Mix yogurt, Parmesan cheese, mayonnaise, milk and garlic powder together in large bowl.

Add pasta and vegetables to yogurt mixture and toss.

Refrigerate at least 2 hours.

Zucchini, Carrot, Grapefruit and Avocado Salad v

Serves 2

1 avocado
1–2 carrots, scraped
2 large zucchinis
1 grapefruit
Vinaigrette
coarsely ground black pepper

Cut the avocado in two and discard the pit. Cut away the outer shell and slice each half in strips.

Using a potato peeler, slice long strips down the length of the carrots and zucchinis, making ribbons.

Cut the grapefruit in two halves and, preferably using a grapefruit knife, carefully cut out segments. Add to the vegetables.

Add enough Vinaigrette to coat the vegetables. Sprinkle with black pepper.

Vegetable Paella v

Serves 2

$1/2$ an eggplant, chopped
salt
1 tbsp olive oil
$1/2$ a small onion, chopped
3 slices each red and green pepper, chopped
$1/2$ a carrot, chopped
1 clove garlic, crushed
$3^1/2$ oz (100g) long-grain rice
1 small tin of chopped tomatoes with herbs
$1/2$ tsp turmeric
coarsely ground black pepper
fresh parsley

Lay the eggplant on a board and cover with salt.
Leave for 20 minutes. Wash and drain.

Heat the olive oil in a large frying pan. Add the
onions and gently sauté until soft.

Add the peppers, eggplant, carrot and garlic,
and stir.

Add the raw rice and the tomatoes, plus
1 cup (300ml) water and the turmeric. Season to
taste.

Bring to the boil, then reduce heat and
simmer until all the water has been absorbed by
the rice.

Serve with a good sprinkling of parsley.

Fava Beans with Parmesan

This works well with plain grilled tuna or swordfish
steaks

$3^1/2$ cups of fresh fava beans
$1/3$ cup extra virgin olive oil
2 garlic cloves, finely chopped
$1/2$ tsp crushed red pepper
salt and freshly ground black pepper
Parmesan or Tuscan Pecorino cheese

Bring a large pot of lightly salted water to a boil.
Add the beans and cook just until the skins loosen,
about 1 minute. Drain and rinse under cold water.
Peel the beans.

Heat the oil, garlic, and red pepper in a
medium skillet over medium high heat until the
garlic is softened, but not browned, about 2
minutes. Add the beans and toss until heated
through and coated with the oil, about 1 minute.
Season to taste with salt and pepper. Transfer into
a serving bowl. Using a vegetable peeler, shave
curls of Pecorino or Parmesan cheese.

Bread

Unbleached White Bread

Makes one large loaf

1 lb unbleached white flour
1 teaspoon easy-bake yeast granules
1 tsp salt
2 tsp sugar
1 tbsp olive oil or butter
1/2 pint warmed water with a splash of milk

Sift the flour into a large bowl, make a well in the center and add the water, milk, yeast, sugar, salt and oil or butter.

Fold the flour over the top and start to incorporate the ingredients. The mixture might feel sticky to start with, but it will soon start to combine.

If the mixture is a little wet, add more flour, a teaspoon at a time.

Once the dough has formed into a ball, turn it onto a floured surface to begin kneading.

Knead the dough, repeatedly bringing the outside to the center, for at least ten minutes; this is hard work, but worth it. When it is ready, put back into your mixing bowl and cover with a clean dish towel to rise. This will take about two hours at room temperature, or you can leave it overnight in the fridge. Don't leave it somewhere too warm – this will kill the yeast.

When the dough has doubled in size, take it out and knead again. This is called "knocking-back" as all the air will go out of it. Do not knead again fully; simply place dough into one large or two smaller greased and floured bread tins. Cover and leave in a warm place, to rise again.

Preheat the oven to 425°F. When the bread dough has doubled in size once again, you are ready to bake your bread.

Bake for 20–30 minutes, or until the bread sounds hollow when tapped on the bottom. If it is not ready, put it back into the oven on the bare shelf, not in the tin, for a few minutes.

Allow to cool completely before slicing.

Desserts

Real Fresh Fruit Gelatin

Makes a large bowlful. A serving is 3 tbsp.

This is incredibly simple, but works with any fruit puree. It is the only way to eat gelatin since store bought versions contain additives, chemicals and colorings.

3 cups fresh fruit puree, not over-sweetened. Works best with strawberries, apricots, mango, pineapple or any combination of these fruits. Make sure the puree is soft but not wet.
1 envelope knox gelatin
1 cup water

Put the gelatin in a cup and mix with a little cold water, to a paste. Add the remaining water.

Place this cup in a bowl or pan of boiling water. Leave for ten minutes, stirring now and again to stop the gelatin clumping. It will dissolve.

When the gelatin is clear, fold immediately into the fruit puree and make sure it is well combined.

Serve with fresh berries or sliced mango. Dust with powdered sugar.

Delicious High-Fiber Fruit Salad

This salad keeps well for several days and is delicious with Greek yogurt or fromage frais. Eat only as a late evening snack, for gut cleanliness.

A serving is 2 tablespoons.

1¹/₃ cups pure apple juice
6 cloves
juice and rind of three oranges
1 cinnamon stick
¹/₂ cup dried apricots
¹/₂ cup dried cranberries
¹/₂ cup dried peaches
¹/₂ cup dried prunes or figs

Put all the ingredients into a heavy-based pan, and simmer on the stove for half an hour.

Remove everything except the liquid, turn up the heat to a steady boil.

Boil until the liquid is reduced by half, approximately. Take out the cloves.

Pour the liquid over the stewed fruits and keep in the refrigerator until needed.

Spiced Poached Pear

This simple dish is an elegant way to finish a calorie-controlled diet and is wonderful to top off a light lunch with friends.

1 whole pear per person
3 cloves
pinch cinnamon
pinch mixed spice
1 glass of red wine
1 tbsp brown sugar per pear

Prepare the pear by slicing the peel off thinly, preserving the stalk and shape of each fruit. Cut a slice off the bottom so the pear will stand upright.

Place the pear carefully in a tall saucepan. Add water until half way up the fruit.

Add the cloves and spices.

Put the lid on the pan and simmer gently for about 30 minutes.

Test with a sharp thin knife, to see that the fruit is soft. If not, continue to poach until it is.

Remove the fruits, place in a serving dish and set aside.

Add the sugar and wine to the liquid, simmer again and when the sugar has dissolved, bring to a bubbling boil. Boil until the liquid has reduced by half.

Pour this spicy liquor over the fruits, sprinkle with grated nutmeg and serve whole, hot or cold, with either home-made chocolate sauce (recipe follows), a spoonful of fromage frais on the side, or a generous spoonful of fresh berries.

Home-Made Chocolate Sauce

I don't use a lot of this, but a spoonful over half
a canned or baked pear makes a delicious and
surprisingly low-calorie sweet dish. Don't make too
much, or you'll be tempted to dip into it!

1 cup dark plain chocolate

2 cups water

$^1/_4$ cup sugar (superfine or Domino's "bar")

$^2/_3$ cup heavy or whipping cream

Put the chocolate into the water, in a pan.

Add the sugar. Bring to the boil and reduce to
a simmer for 15 minutes.

Remove from the heat and stir in the cream.

Refrigerate until needed.

And Finally . . .

It is so wonderful to feel your stomach flat. You have finally got into a whole new way of eating and caring for yourself, and I hope you think it is worth it.

You might still have a way to go. Maybe you have several pounds to lose and it seems daunting. Don't think of it that way. When you fall out of the habit, or you have gone back to your old ways, get back on track by doing the following:

1 Start again – forget what you have done.
2 Remind yourself of your bottom line.
3 Have you gone to the person whom you told your new plan to?
  Call him or her—don't wallow, and have a nice chat.
4 Get out and exercise.
5 Congratulate yourself—for each simple thing you do on your midline.

Respect yourself, respect others and respect food. Above all, never fall into the trap of believing the hype about not being able to lose weight after forty or never having a flat stomach after a baby. You will. Remember your bottom line and . . .

Good luck!